AF577169

ILLUSTRATED GUIDE TO THE CENTRAL NERVOUS SYSTEM

Kazuaki Sugiura, M.D.
Head, Dept. of Neurosurgery
Tokyo Rohsai Hospital

Grant A. Robinson, Ph.D.
Postdoctoral Fellow
College of Medicine
University of Arizona

Douglas G. Stuart, Ph.D.
Professor of Physiology
College of Medicine
University of Arizona

English Translation by:
Eisaku Kanazawa, M.D.
Department of Anatomy
Dental School at Matsudo
Nippon University

Ishiyaku EuroAmerica, Inc.
St. Louis • Tokyo

Book Editor: Gregory Hacke, D.C.

FIRST EDITION

Ishiyaku EuroAmerica, Inc.
716 Hanley Industrial Court, St. Louis, Missouri 63144

Library of Congress Catalogue Card Number 88-81243

Sugiura, Kazuaki
Robinson, Grant A.
Stuart, Douglas G.
Illustrated Guide to the Central Nervous System

ISBN 0-912791-45-4

Ishiyaku EuroAmerica, Inc.
St. Louis • Tokyo

Composition by TSI Graphics, Inc., St. Louis, Missouri 63144
Printed in Japan

PREFACE

This work is a translation of a very popular book among Japanese students of neurosurgery and neurology. Dr. Sugiura received his M.D. from the Nippon Medical School, in 1965, neurosurgical training at the University of Edinburgh (1972) and has been the Head of the Department of Neurosurgery at Tokyo Rohsai Hospital since 1977. This book was prompted by Dr. Sugiura's former students who valued the concise yet complete format of his lectures and illustrations. Dr. Sugiura designed this book to refresh medical students' and house officers' minds and as a primer dealing with clinical aspects of the brain's structural and functional relationships: an excellent approach for allied health students as well.

At the University of Arizona, as at several others in the U.S.A., neuroanatomy is now a popular course for upper-division undergraduates majoring in exercise and sport science, nursing, psychology, and speech and hearing science. Our neuroscience group also teaches human neuroanatomy as part of a continuing-education neuroscience course taken by teachers of special education, members of the allied health professions (particularly nurses and occupational and physical therapists) and members of the lay public who are active in clinical-neural organizations. Dr. Sugiura's approach (including a historical perspective) should appeal to all such students.

Whatever the reader's goal, it is hoped that this work will stimulate the pursuit of more specific and detailed literature on the fascinating topic of human neuroanatomy and its equally interesting comparative counterparts.

In this translation, an attempt has been made to retain the freshness and intimacy of Dr. Sugiura's original work while, at the same time, updating selected areas. We would like to thank Dr. Joachim Seeger, Professor of Radiology, for his help with the section on computerized tomography and Dr. Colin Bamford, Associate Professor of Neurology, for his careful review of the clinical sections and for providing a clinical perspective.

Grant A. Robinson, Ph.D.
Douglas G. Stuart, Ph.D.
Department of Physiology
College of Medicine
University of Arizona
Tucson, Arizona

CLINICAL PERSPECTIVE

Early in my training as a medical student, I became clearly aware that the rate that I was acquiring information was more rapid when I was studying from illustrated textbooks. I noticed that the retention of this material was better and my performance on examinations superior.

There is probably no medical field that lends itself more to study by means of illustration than that of the nervous system. Dr. Sugiura has effectively accomplished the goal of preparing such a text. His illustrations are accurate and the detail is simple yet appropriate for the point that is being conveyed at that time.

The text is sufficiently concise to allow a reasonably motivated medical student the opportunity to cover this course in the three to four week time frame typically allotted to a neurology or neurosurgery clerkship. The text would clearly be an excellent orientation for the first year Neurology or Neurosurgery Resident in the first few months of their ward rotation.

Whereas the illustrations are excellent and the clinical points concise, the text does not pretend to expound on the latest technological developments in diagnosis or treatment. The author, at times, recommends management that may be sensible economically, yet may subject the patient to a slightly increased risk of complication, which should be avoided considering the medico-legal climate of the United States. These points have been addressed in the text.

Colin R. Bamford, M.D.
Associate Professor of Neurology
College of Medicine
University of Arizona
Tucson, Arizona

CONTENTS

I. STRUCTURE AND FUNCTION

FEATURES OF THE CENTRAL NERVOUS SYSTEM (CNS)

ANATOMICAL ORIENTATION

Most anatomical descriptions in this text are referenced to standard anatomical position. There are several pitfalls inherent in some descriptions. For example, the small mounds on the posterior aspect of the brain stem are called the superior and inferior colliculi, even though their relative positions could be described as rostral on the neural axis for the superior set and caudal on the axis for the inferior set.

OVERALL FUNCTION

The human body continuously reacts to changes of internal or external circumstances (stimuli) by means of muscular contraction and glandular secretion. During these processes, the role of the CNS is to integrate stimulus-induced sensory information with ongoing central activity in order to achieve appropriate effector outputs.

The nervous system (central and peripheral) can be divided into several categories, based on function and location (Tables 1, 2). It is essential to understand these basic subdivisions.

DEVELOPMENT

Development of the nervous system (Figs. 1–3) begins on the embryo's 16th or 17th day. First, a longitudinal band of cell proliferation on the dorsal median line of the ectoderm thickens to form the neural plate (2-A). This structure thickens and folds inward to become the neural groove (1, 2-B). At about 22 days (1), the neural groove deepens and separates from the dorsal surface to form the neural tube centrally, still remaining in the cranial and caudal portions. The cranial portion of the tube is completed at about 26 days and the caudal portion at 28 days, forming a complete neural tube. At the same time, the cranial structures begin to swell and form a primitive brain by the end of the third month (Fig. 3).

Somites which are derived from mesoderm begin to develop (Fig. 1) in a cranial to caudal sequence. By 30 days, they comprise 42–44 pairs from which most of the body's skeleton and musculature are derived. The spinal column is formed by fusion of bilateral somites in the median plane. A disturbance of this fusion process may result in spina bifida. It might also become a meningocele or myelomeningocele and is usually accompanied by an incomplete neural tube formation.

Table 1. DIVISIONS OF THE NERVOUS SYSTEM BASED ON FUNCTION

somatic nervous system	general sensory nerves general motor nerves	largely voluntary and automatic actions
autonomic (visceral) nervous system	visceral sensory visceral smooth muscle cardiac tissue glandular muscle	largely involuntary actions

Table 2. DIVISIONS OF THE NERVOUS SYSTEM BASED ON LOCATION

central nervous system	cerebrum, diencephalon, midbrain, pons, cerebellum, medulla oblongata, spinal cord (The midbrain, pons and medulla are collectively called the brain stem.)
peripheral nervous system	cranial nerves 12 pairs spinal nerves 31 pairs (cervical, 8 pairs; thoracic, 12 pairs; lumbar, 5 pairs; sacral, 5 pairs; coccygeal, 1 pair)

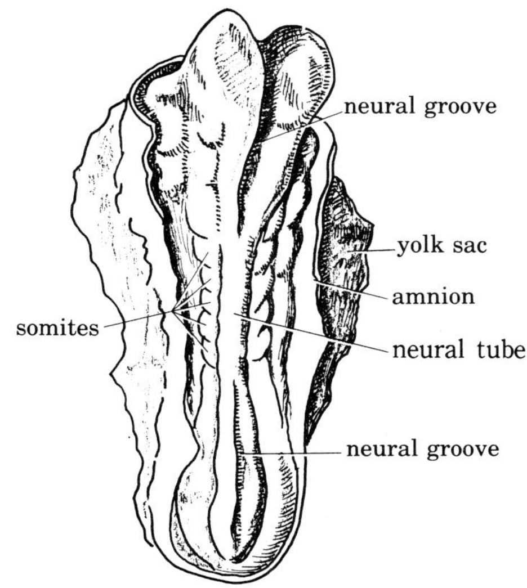

Fig. 1 The embryo at about 22 days after fertilization.
A dorsal view of the neural tube, which has already formed in the central part, and connects rostrally and caudally to the neural groove.

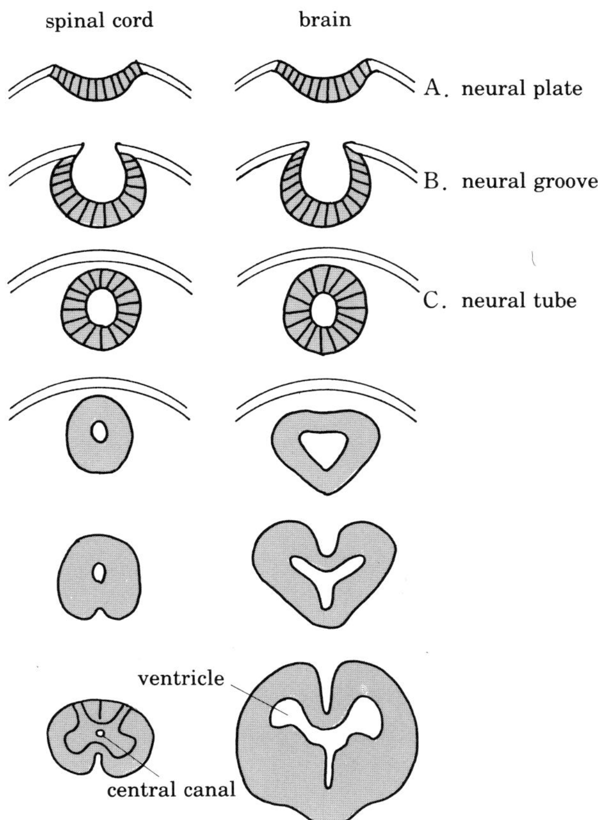

Fig. 2 Progressive development of the central nervous system.
The central canal of the spinal cord and the ventricles of the brain are homologous structures. The complex shapes of the ventricles result from the relatively unequal development of different parts of the brain (cerebrum, cerebellum, midbrain, diencephalon, pons, etc.).

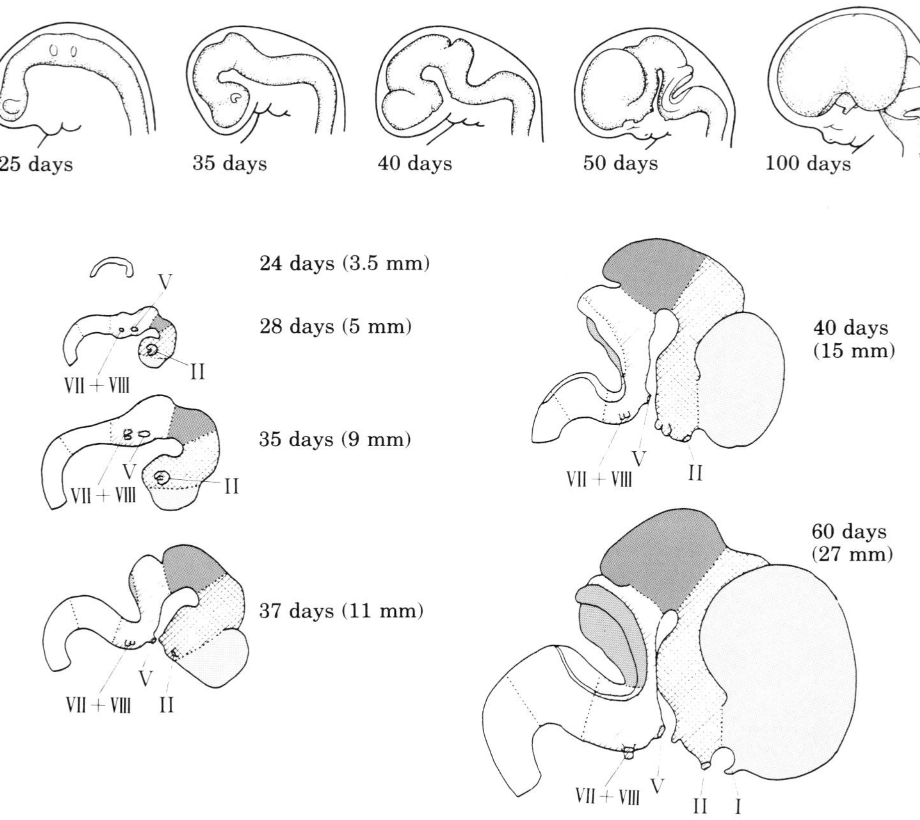

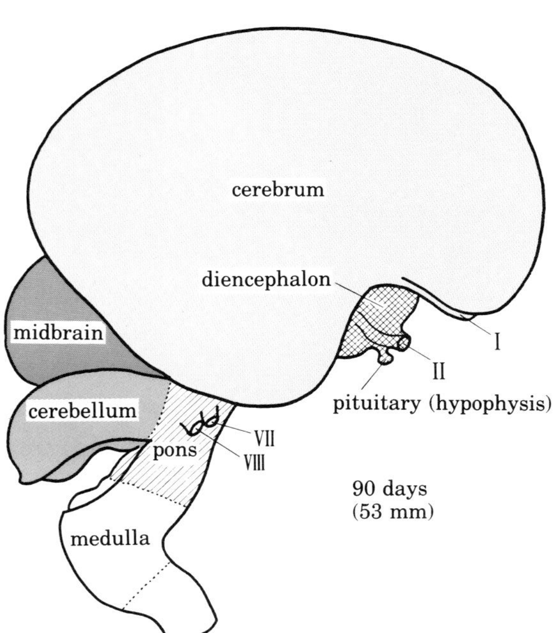

Fig. 3 Relative development of selected parts of the brain. Approximations of embryo age (body lengths are shown in parentheses). Roman numerals indicate cranial nerves I-VIII (after Hoffstetter). The diagrams are twice actual size except for those in the top row which are further magnified to reveal detail. The brain is formed by a tremendous swelling at the cranial end of the neural tube. Foldings (into gyri and sulci) on the surface of the cerebrum do not appear until the middle of pregnancy. The developed human brain has about a hundred billion neurons, a number that does not increase after birth. Accordingly, the embryonic brain must generate more than 250 thousand neurons per minute during periods of rapid development.

CELLULAR ELEMENTS

Nervous tissue is composed of neurons and glial cells. The former are classified into three categories: motoneurons, sensory neurons and interneurons. Fig. 4 is a diagram of a typical neuron drawn at 250 times its real size. The impulse generated near the cell body is conducted along the axon at a velocity ranging from less than 1 to 120 meters per second. The velocity depends on the diameter of the axon and the presence or absence of a myelin sheath. Wider axons have faster conduction velocities because of their lower resistance to longitudinal current flow. Similarly, the thicker the myelin sheaths, the faster the conduction velocity.

Neuroglia perform a variety of functions for neurons such as stabilizing their connections with one another, providing nutrition from the blood, absorbing waste products and forming myelin sheaths for neuronal axons. Glial cells are divided into three types: astrocytes, oligodendrocytes and microglia. The former two, like neurons, originate from ectoderm but microglia are derived from mesoderm. Gliomas, the most frequent form of brain tumor, are usually composed of astrocytes.

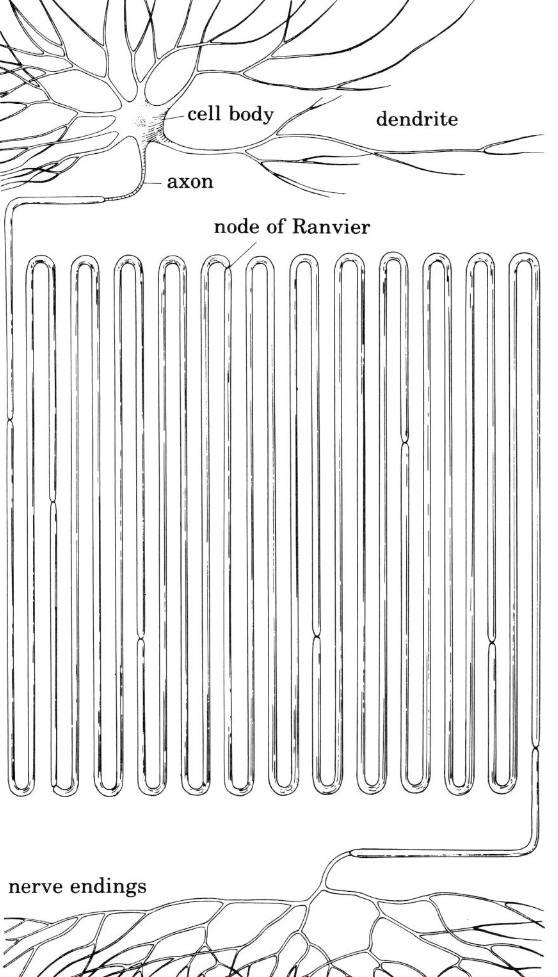

Fig. 4 Structure of a typical neuron.

Axon length ranges from about 1 m to 1 cm. Axon terminals form as many as 1000 synapses with other neurons. About 50% of all axons are wrapped by myelin sheaths which increase their conduction velocity.

GROSS ARCHITECTURE

Figure 5 shows the gross architecture of the CNS. It consists of the cerebrum (5-1), diencephalon (5-2), mesencephalon (5-3), pons (5-4), cerebellum (5-6), medulla oblongata (5-5) and spinal cord (5-7) from top (rostral) to bottom (caudal). These names and locations must be memorized to understand the following descriptions of neurological symptoms and diseases.

The diencephalon cannot be seen from the outside. It is located at the center of the brain, surrounded by the cerebrum. The diencephalon, midbrain, pons and medulla oblongata comprise the brain stem, a useful term when describing actions of the reticular formation and the effects of lesions on selected structures.

The CNS is completely protected by the skeleton, the medulla and more rostral structures within the cranium, and the spinal cord within the spinal column. An important opening is the foramen magnum (8-6, 10-24, 19-B) where, as described later, tonsilar herniation of the cerebellum can occur.

Additional foramina in the cranial base provide passage for 12 cranial nerves and intervertebral foramina are available for the spinal nerves.

The spinal cord ends caudally as the conus medullaris at the level of the first lumbar vertebra (5-A). Lumbar puncture (to sample cerebrospinal fluid) is carried out at the level of a line (Jacoby's) connecting both iliac crests in order not to damage the spinal cord (5-B).

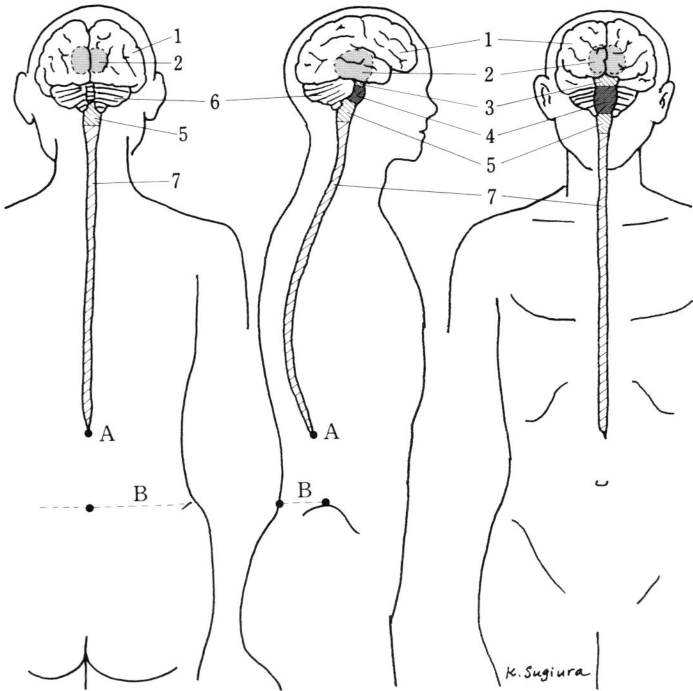

Fig. 5 Gross architecture of the CNS.

1. cerebrum (telencephalon)
2. diencephalon
3. midbrain
4. pons
5. medulla
6. cerebellum
7. spinal cord
   A. caudal end of spinal cord
   B. Jacoby's line

2. PROTECTIVE COVERINGS OF THE BRAIN

SCALP

The scalp serves to cushion the brain somewhat (Fig. 6). However, the scalp's skin (6–1) and subcutaneous tissue (6–2) are not particularly resistant to externally applied forces. They are densely vascularized. Consequently, the scalp has both the disadvantage of being prone to lacerating wounds and bleeding, and the advantage of preventing brain infection and promoting fast healing. Internal to the subcutaneous tissue, is the galea (6–3), the strongest tissue in the scalp for resisting external forces. During craniotomy, it is reflected using Pean's forceps. After surgery, tight suturing of the galea is necessary to prevent splitting of the scalp. The periosteum lies under the scalp, but unlike long-bone periosteum, it does not produce bone well.

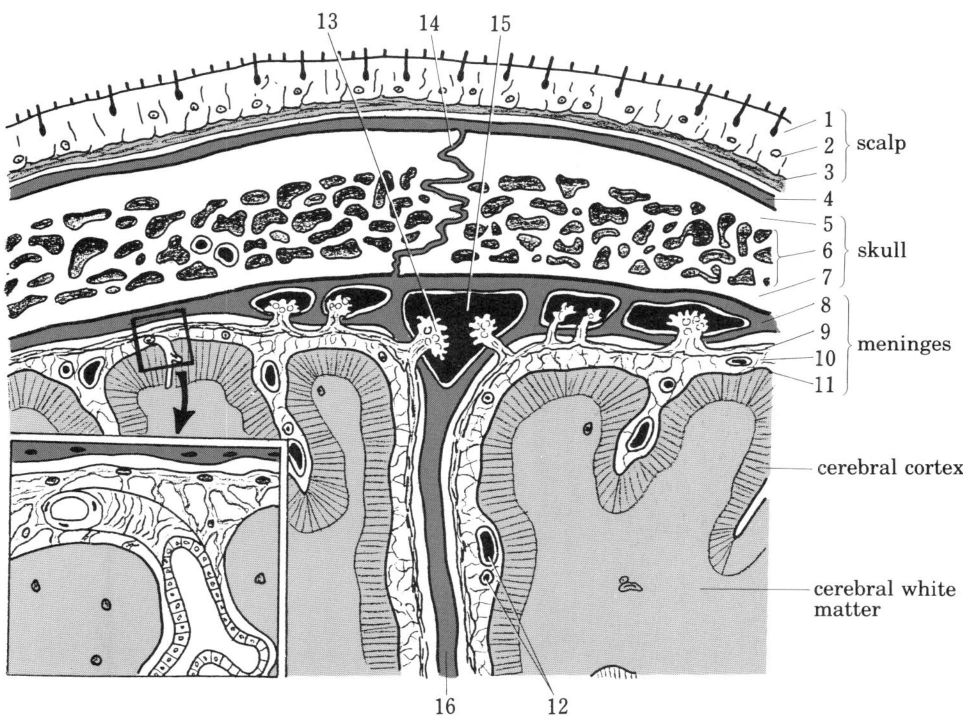

Fig. 6 Protective coverings and structures of the brain.

1. skin
2. subcutaneous tissue
3. galea
4. periosteum
5. outer table
6. diploe
7. inner table
8. dura mater
9. arachnoid
10. subarachnoid space
11. pia mater
12. artery and vein
13. arachnoid granulation
14. sagittal suture
15. superior sagittal sinus
16. falx cerebri

SKULL

The skull consists of 23 bones of 15 different types (Table 3). They protect the brain by forming a thick wall with complicated sutures. In addition, they have several foramina for the passage of cranial nerves, blood vessels and the medulla.

Fig. 7 provides lateral and superior views of the infant skull. There are two fontanelles, anterior (7–6) and posterior (7–8). These are used both for monitoring intracranial pressure and for subdural puncture in infants.

Figs. 9–10 present some of the innumerable terms for bones, sutures and foramina. Before memorizing them, it is valuable to visualize their corresponding structures as three-dimensional images in relation to the brain's internal arrangements and external landmarks (e.g., note the external acoustic meatus and orbital cavity in Fig. 8).

The anterior cranial fossa (8–2), adjacent to the frontal lobe, is at the level of the upper orbital wall. The middle cranial fossa (8–4), next to the temporal lobe, is at the level of the external acoustic meatus. The posterior cranial fossa (8–5), adjacent to the cerebellum, is located a few centimeters below this meatus. The different levels of the three cranial fossae should be noted. Similarly, the level and location of the sella turcica (8–8), its encased hypophysis (pituitary gland) (8–7) and the adjacent optic nerve also deserve emphasis.

Terms for the many foramina in the cranial base should be memorized in relation to their corresponding cranial nerves. However, it is difficult to understand these relationships in two-dimensional diagrams. Direct observation of the skull for about an hour is required in order to gain a three-dimensional understanding. The sagittal, coronal and lambdoid sutures are clinically important for differentiating fractures of skull bones and in understanding craniosynostosis, caused by an early fusion of sutures, and with their subsequent separation by increased intracranial pressure.

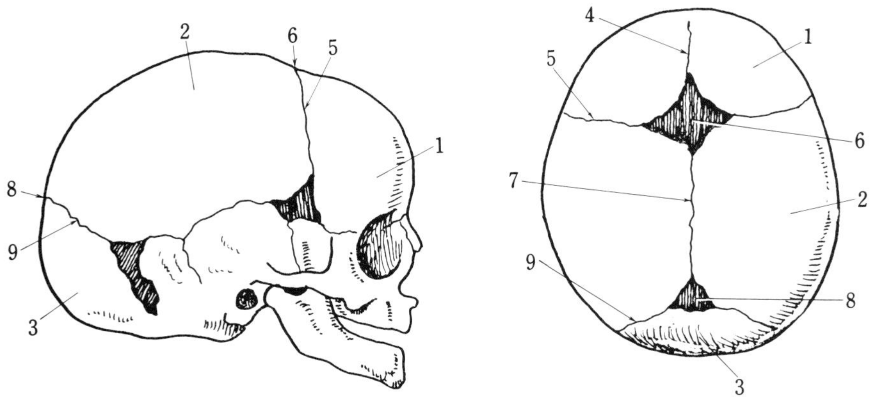

Fig. 7 The skull at birth

1. frontal bone
2. parietal bone
3. occipital bone
4. frontal suture
5. coronal suture
6. anterior fontanelle
7. sagittal suture
8. posterior fontanelle
9. lambdoid suture

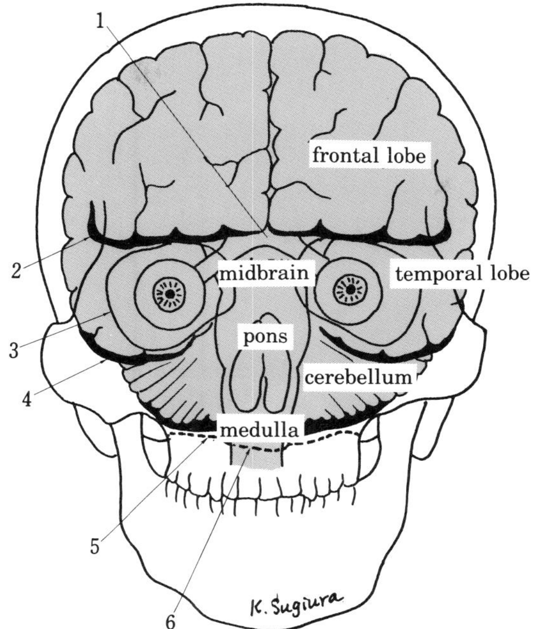

A Frontal view

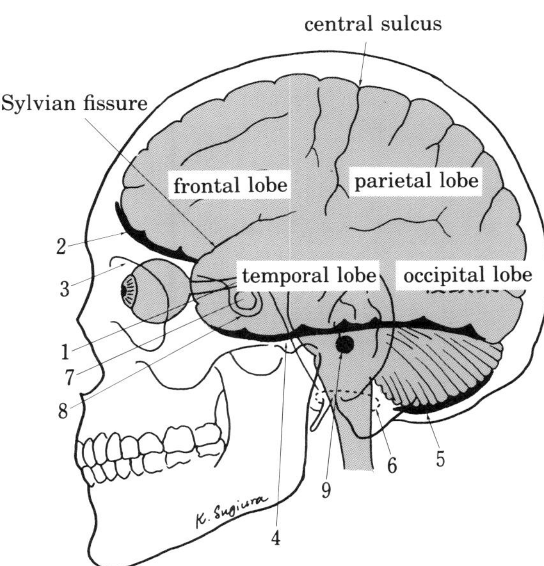

B Lateral view

Fig. 8 Brain-skull relationships.

1. optic nerve
2. anterior cranial fossa
3. orbital cavity
4. middle cranial fossa
5. posterior cranial fossa
6. foramen magnum
7. hypophysis
8. sella turcica
9. external acoustic meatus

Note: There are pronounced differences in the heights of the anterior, middle and posterior cranial fossae. This figure explains cerebrospinal fluid flow from the nose and ear and how subcutaneous hemorrhage at the orbital cavity level or mastoid process can occur when the base of the skull is fractured. The foramen magnum is clinically important as a key location for herniation of the cerebellar tonsils.

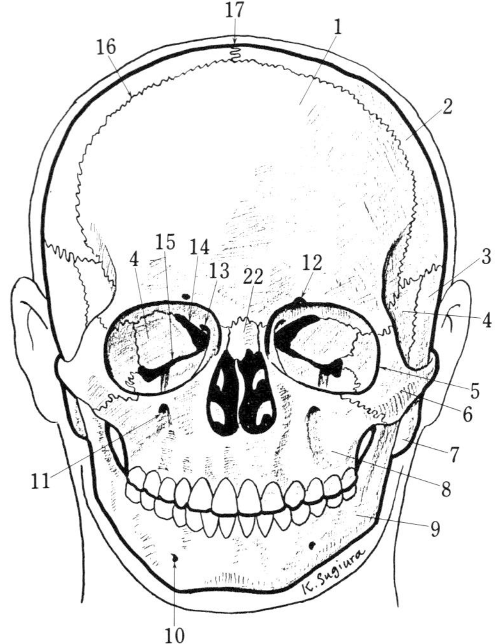

A. Frontal view

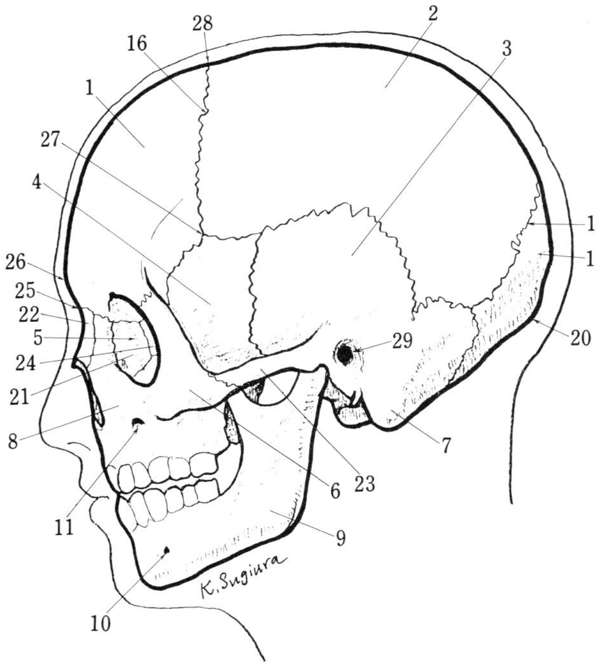

B. Lateral view

Fig. 9 External landmarks of the skull.

1. frontal bone
2. parietal bone
3. temporal bone
4. sphenoid bone
5. orbital cavity
6. zygomatic bone
7. mastoid process
8. maxilla
9. mandible
10. mental foramen
11. infra-orbital foramen
12. supra-orbital foramen
13. optic canal
14. superior orbital fissure
15. inferior orbital fissure
16. coronal suture
17. sagittal suture
18. lambdoid suture
19. occipital bone
20. external occipital protuberance (inion)
21. lacrimal bone
22. nasal bone
23. zygomatic arch
24. ethmoid bone
25. nasion
26. glabella
27. pterion
28. bregma
29. external auditory meatus

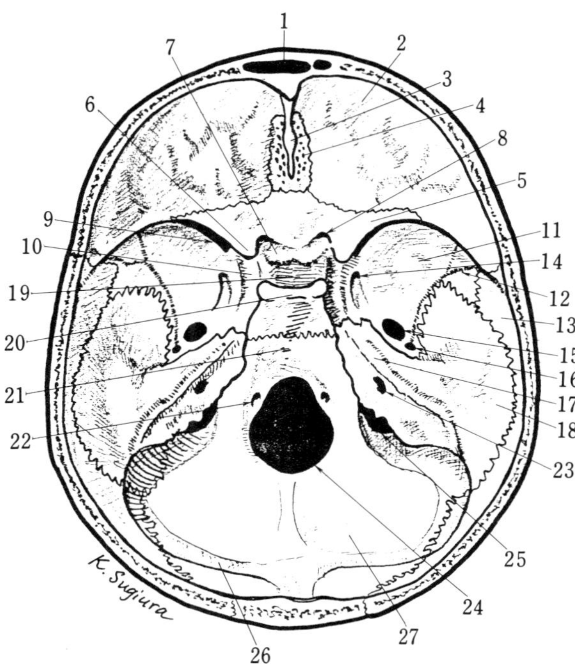

A. internal view of the base of the skull

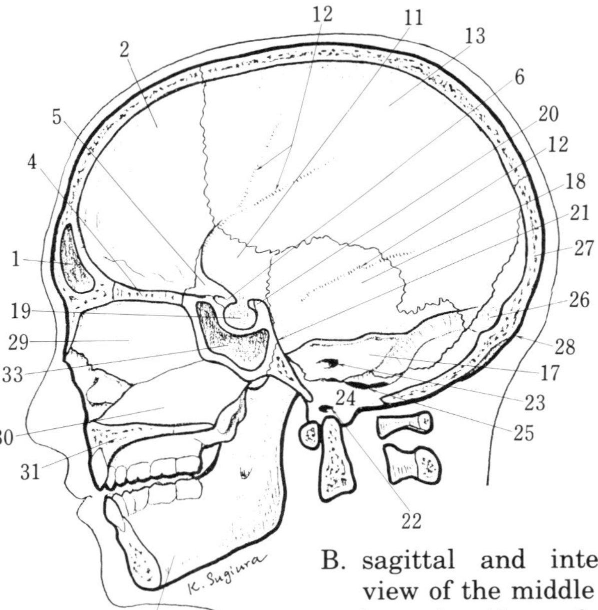

B. sagittal and internal view of the middle and lateral sides of the skull

Fig. 10 Internal landmarks of the skull.

1. frontal sinus
2. frontal bone
3. crista galli
4. cribriform plate
5. lesser wing of the sphenoid bone
6. anterior clinoid process
7. tuberculum sellae
8. optic canal
9. superior orbital fissure
10. carotid groove
11. greater wing of the sphenoid bone
12. groove of the middle meningeal artery
13. parietal bone
14. foramen rotundum
15. foramen ovale
16. foramen spinosum
17. petrous part of the temporal bone
18. squamous part of the temporal bone
19. sella turcica
20. dorsum sellae
21. clivus
22. hypoglossal canal
23. internal acoustic canal
24. foramen magnum
25. jugular foramen
26. groove for the transverse sinus
27. occipital bone
28. inion
29. perpendicular plate of the ethmoid bone
30. vomer
31. maxilla
32. mandible
33. sphenoidal sinus

RADIOGRAPHY OF THE SKULL

Since Rontgen discovered the X-ray in 1895, countless X-ray films have been taken on a world-wide basis. Obviously, this technique has been of the utmost importance for the examination of innumerable diseases. However, it is not completely without risk to the human body, necessitating the continued updating of equipment and radiographic procedures. Furthermore, the correct reading of X-ray images requires mastery of basic anatomy, normal variations and anticipated pathological findings (Table 3, 4).

In a radiograph, three-dimensional structures of the head are projected onto two-dimensional flat film so that the skull's bones overlap each other. To read a film, the direction of projection must always be kept in mind. For example, the images of Figs. 11–13 are very different, even though they have the same sagittal projection. Recognition of the following features of X-ray films considerably facilitates their correct interpretation:

1. The form and shape of the skull
2. The thickness of various bones
3. The sutures, grooves for blood vessels and potential fractures
4. The presence or absence of calcification
5. Potential abnormalities of the sella turcica
6. The location of the cranial base and facial bones, observed in relation to the paranasal sinuses and mastoid cells

MEMORANDUM

After all, to accomplish your studies, you should strive earnestly for a long time, not being tired, not being lazy and constantly with great effort.

Norinaga Motoori
(Japanese philosopher in the 18th century)

Medicine begins, exists and ends with the patient.

William Osler

Examining my body is a waste of time. I do not want a needless examination. But, in tears, my wife asked me to see a doctor. So I made up my mind to have it done. Please examine my blood and urine as if they were my wife's tears.

Ougai Mori
(Japanese doctor and author in the 19th century)

I can even study in a barn, if there are test tubes, a Bunsen burner and blotting papers.

Paul Ehrlich

Table 3. BONES FORMING THE SKULL AND THEIR CHECK POINTS

frontal bone (1)	superior margin of orbital cavity, frontal sinus, coronal suture
parietal bone (2)	sagittal suture
temporal bone (2)	petrous part—internal acoustic canal, external acoustic meatus, foramen lacerum mastoid process—mastoid air cells, sigmoid sinus
occipital bone (1)	internal occipital protuberance, external occipital protuberance (inion), foramen magnum, transverse sinus, lambdoid suture
sphenoid bone (1)	lesser wing—anterior clinoid process, optic canal, superior orbital fissure greater wing—foramen ovale, foramen rotundum, foramen spinosum body—sella turcica, dorsum sellae, posterior clinoid process, sphenoidal sinus
ethmoid bone (1)	ethmoidal plate, crista galli, ethmoidal sinus
maxillary bone (2)	maxillary sinus, hard palate, inferior surface of orbital cavity
zygomatic bone (2)	zygomatic arch, lateral margin of orbital cavity
palatine bone (2)	
vomer (1)	
nasal bone (2)	
lacrimal bone (2)	
mandible (1)	
inferior turbinate (2)	
hyoid bone (1)	

(1) and (2) denote unpaired and paired bones, respectively.

Table 4. FORAMINA AND CANALS OF THE SKULL, THEIR NERVES AND BLOOD VESSELS OF PASSAGE

optic foramen—optic nerve (II), ophthalmic artery
foramen rotundum—second branch of trigeminal nerve (maxillary nerve; V-2)
foramen ovale—third branch of trigeminal nerve (mandibular nerve; V-3)
foramen spinosum—middle meningeal artery
foramen lacerum—superficial and deep petrosal nerve, internal carotid artery
foramen jugulare—internal jugular vein, glossopharyngeal nerve (IX), vagus nerve (X), accessory nerve (XI)
hypoglossal foramen—hypoglossal nerve (XII)
internal acoustic canal—facial nerve (VII), vestibulo-cochlear nerve (VIII), artery of the internal ear
external acoustic meatus
foramen magnum—medulla oblongata, vertebral artery, accessory nerve (XI)
superior orbital fissure—oculomotor nerve (III), trochlear nerve (IV), first branch of trigeminal nerve (V-1), abducens nerve (VI)
inferior orbital fissure—second branch of the trigeminal nerve (V-2)

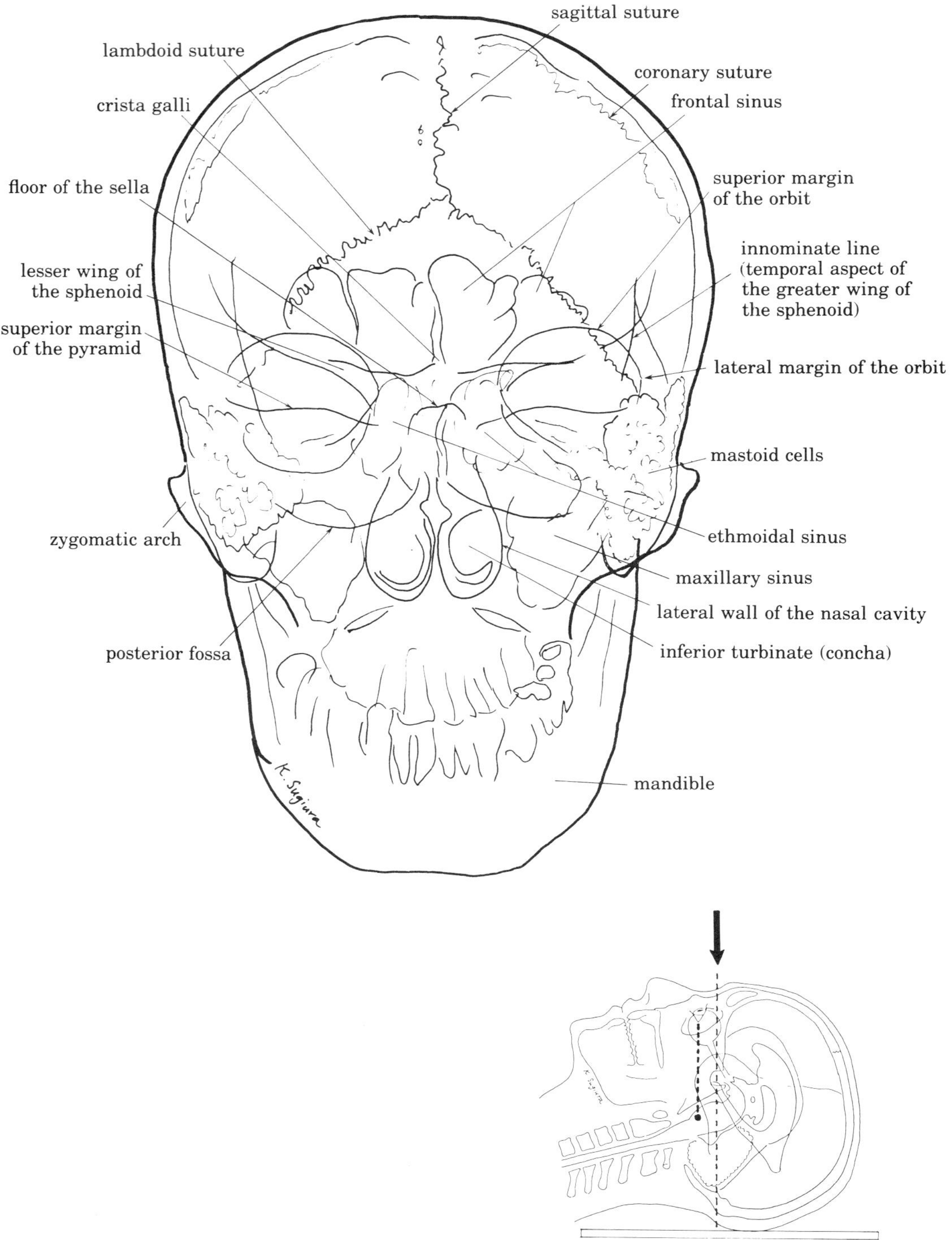

Fig. 11A Normal antero-posterior view.

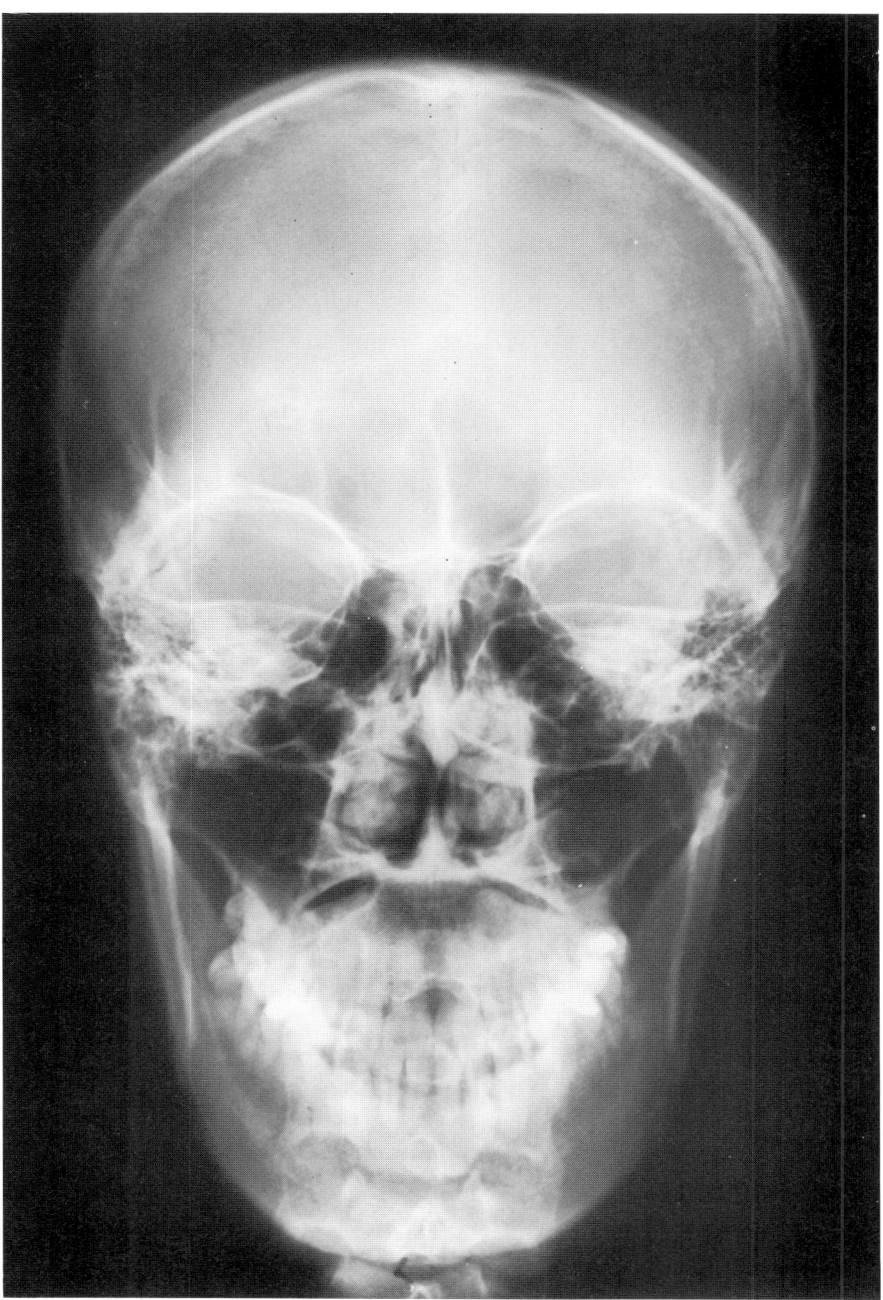

Fig. 11B Normal antero-posterior view.

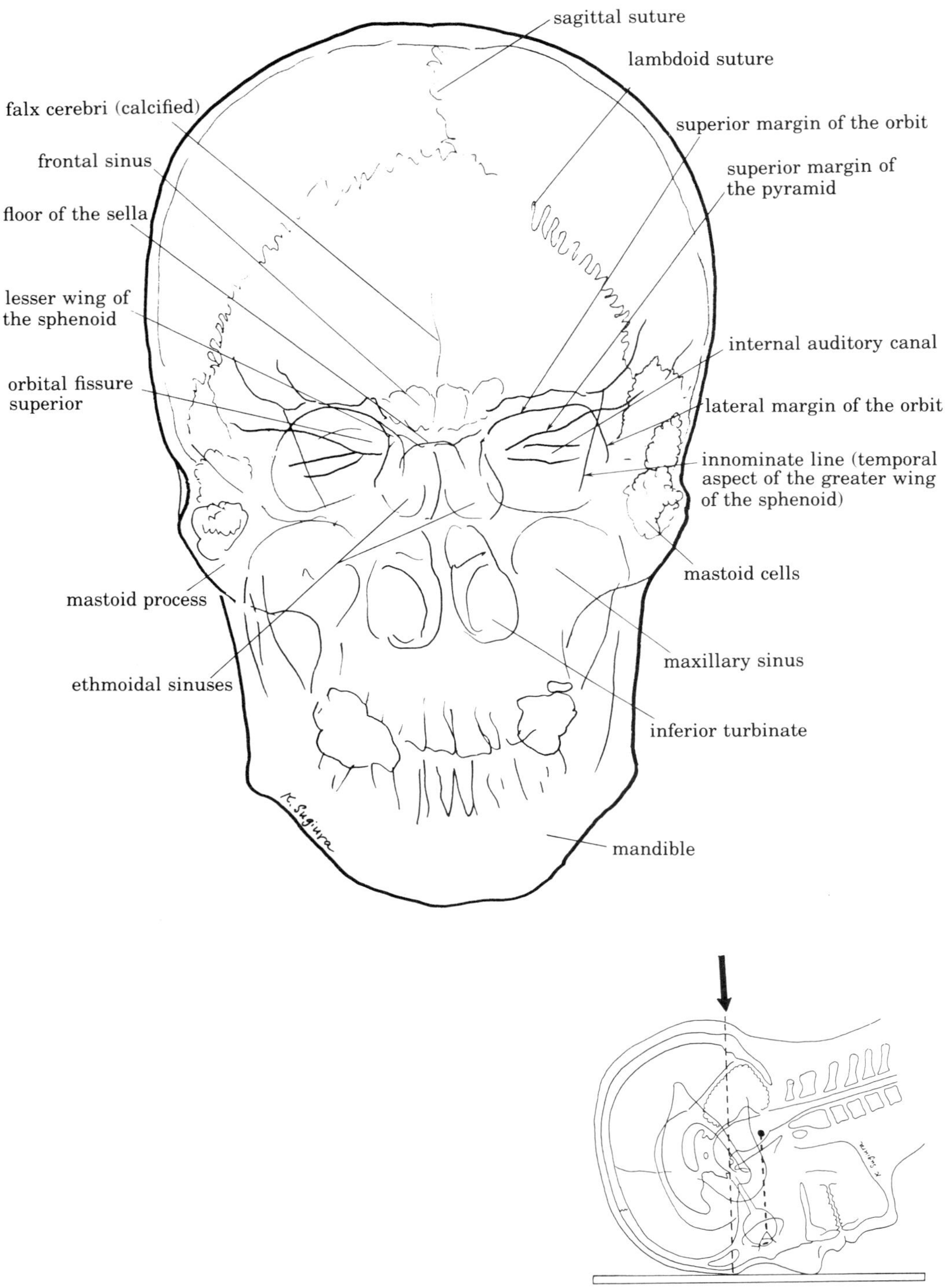

sagittal suture
lambdoid suture
falx cerebri (calcified)
superior margin of the orbit
frontal sinus
superior margin of the pyramid
floor of the sella
lesser wing of the sphenoid
internal auditory canal
orbital fissure superior
lateral margin of the orbit
innominate line (temporal aspect of the greater wing of the sphenoid)
mastoid cells
mastoid process
maxillary sinus
ethmoidal sinuses
inferior turbinate
mandible

Fig. 12A Normal postero-anterior view.

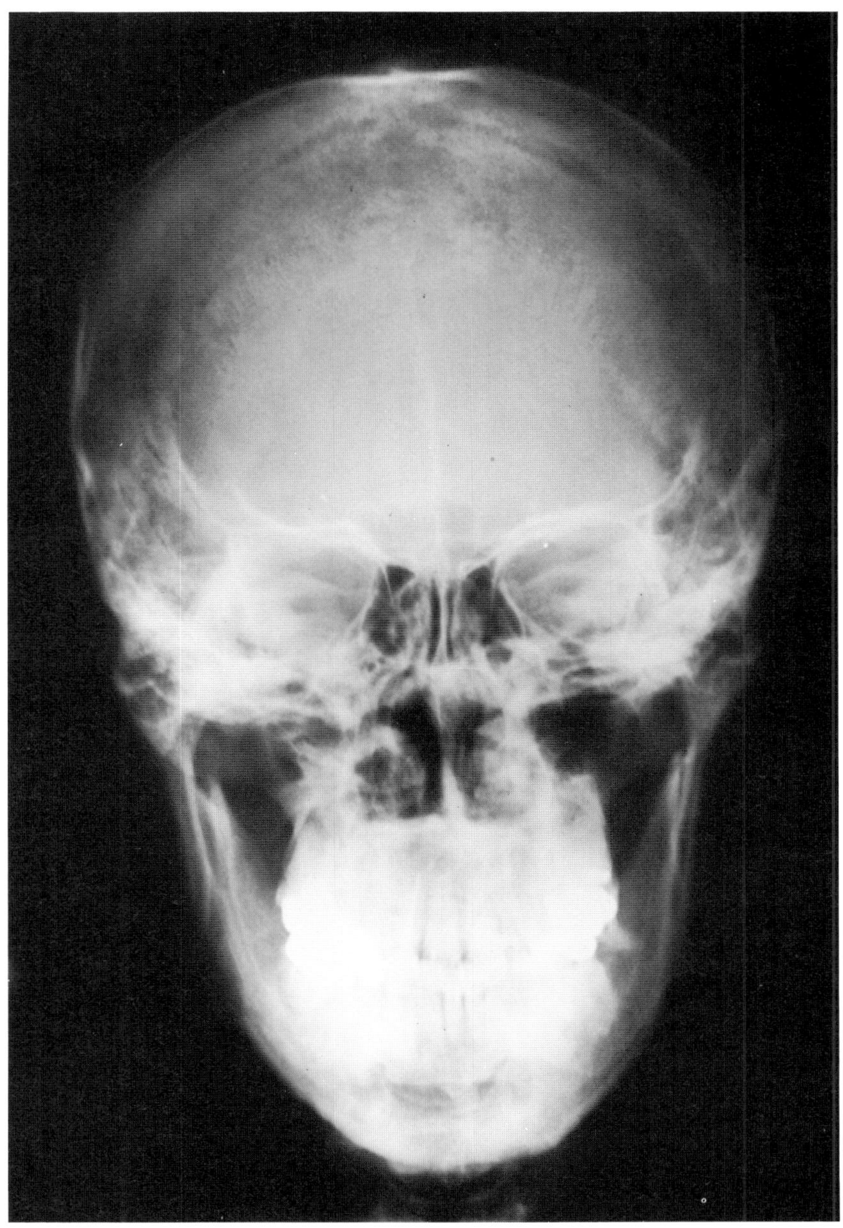

Fig. 12B Normal postero-anterior view.

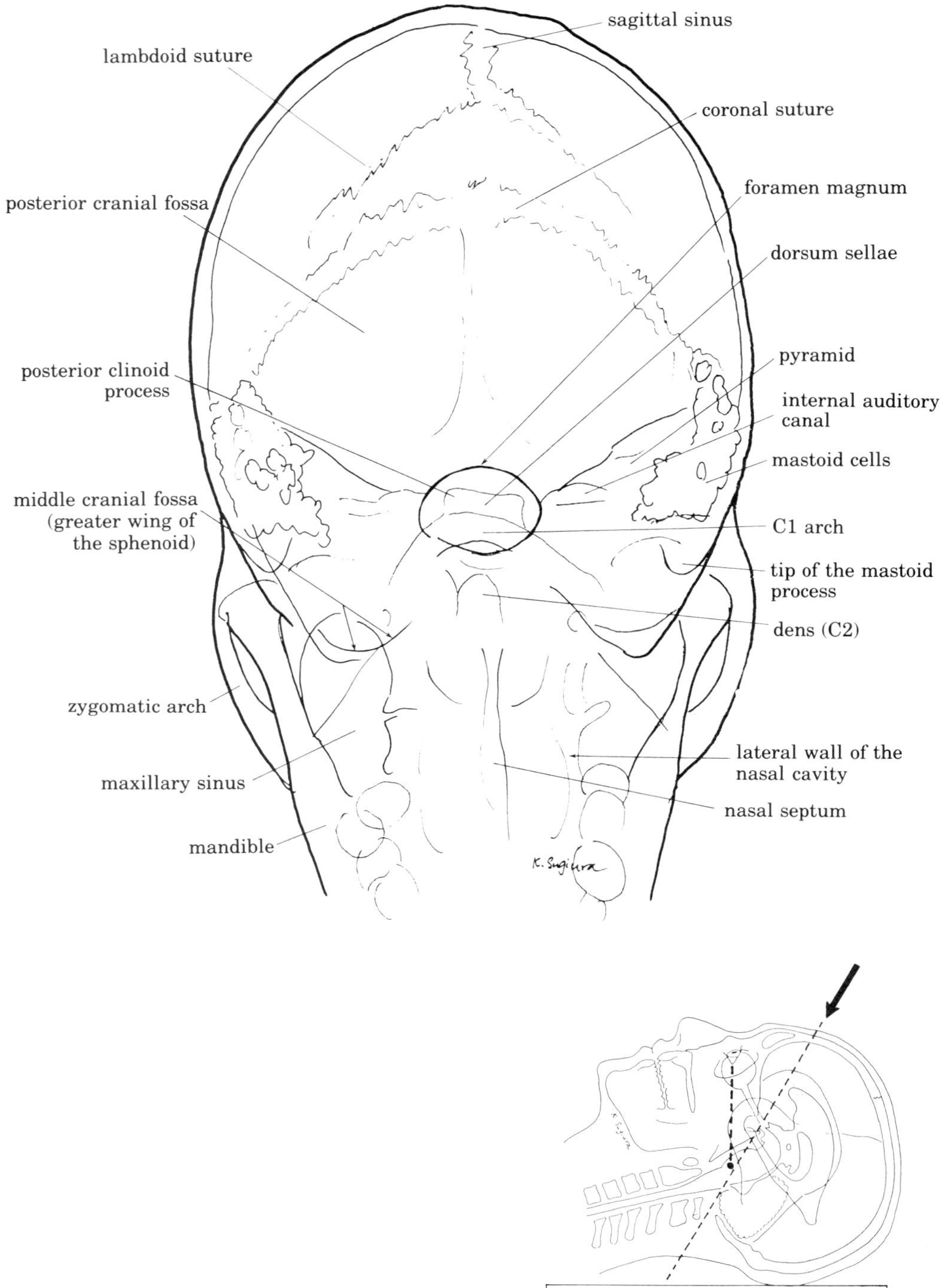

Fig. 13A Normal Towne's view.

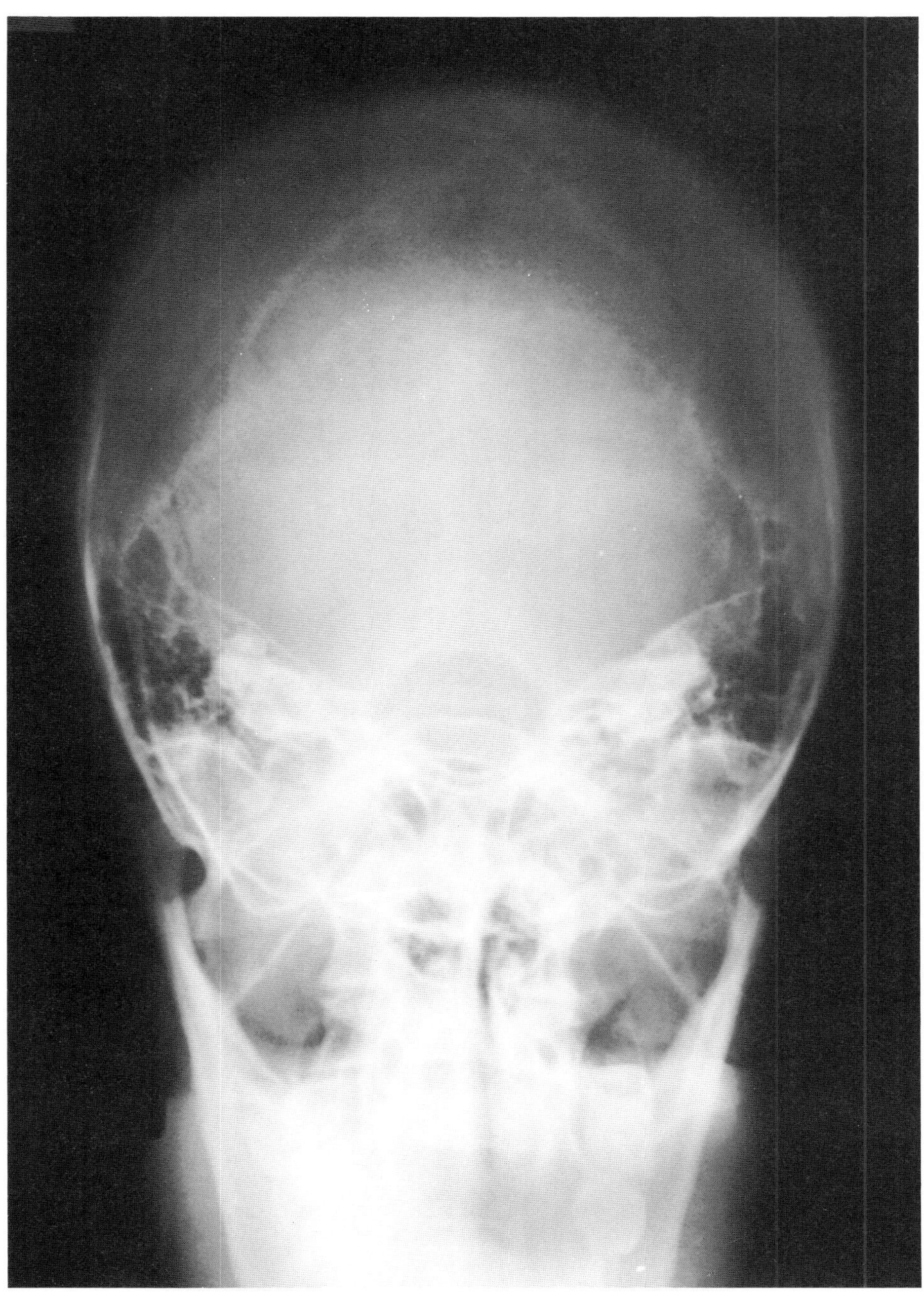

Fig. 13B Normal Towne's view.

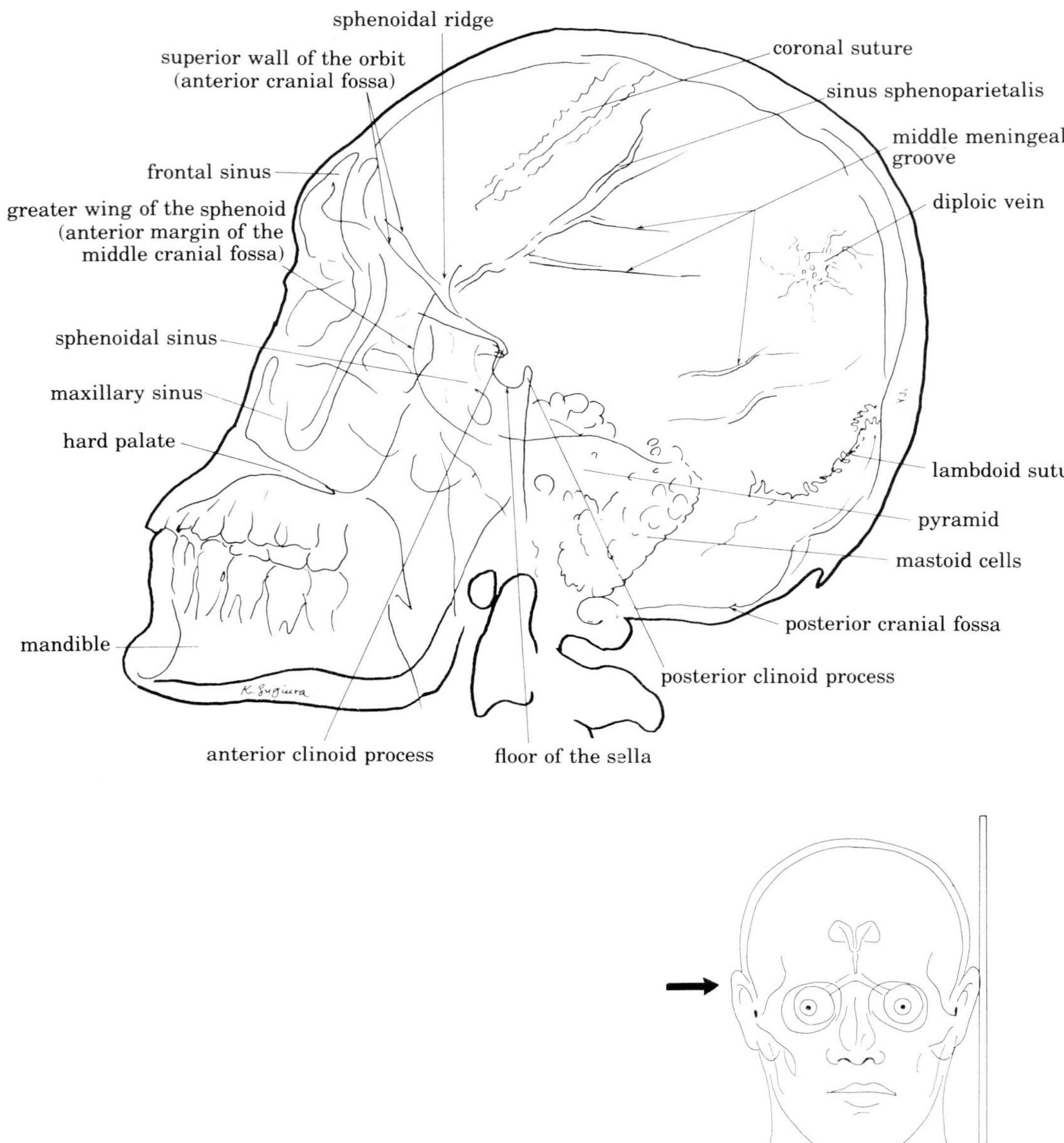

Fig. 14A Normal lateral view.

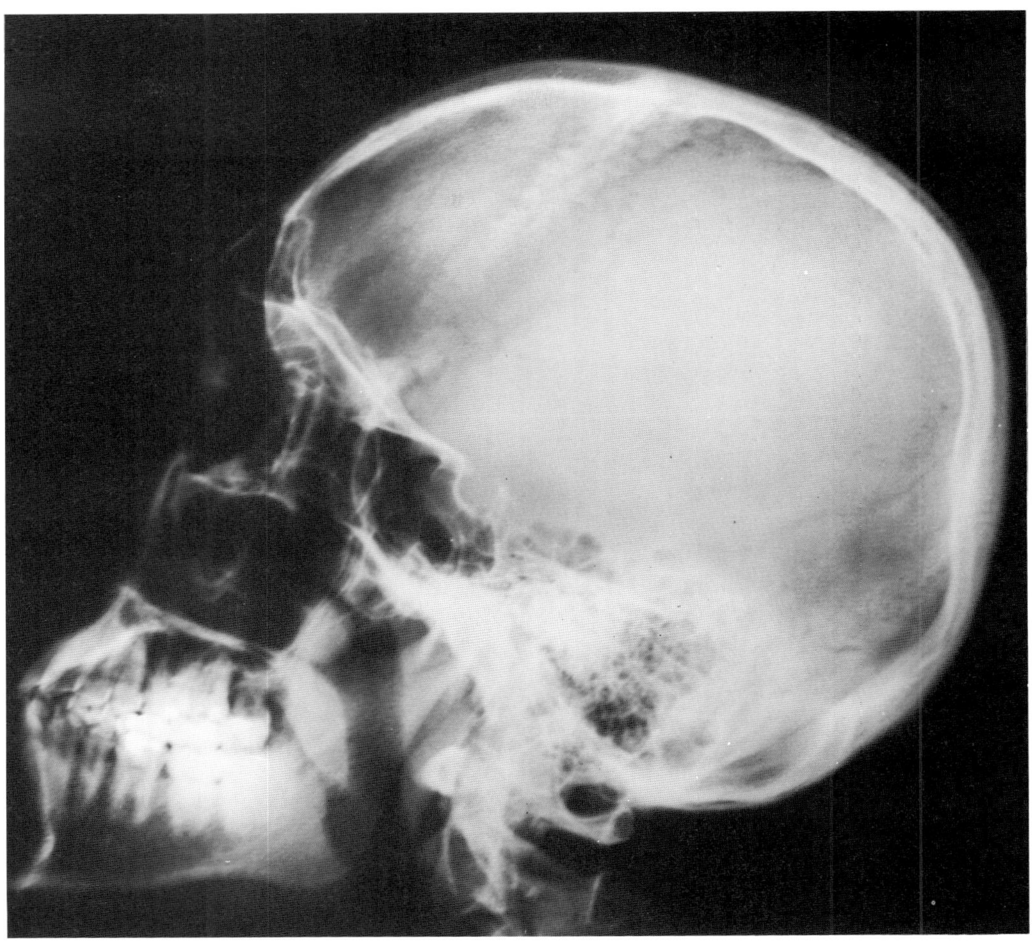

Fig. 14B Normal lateral view.

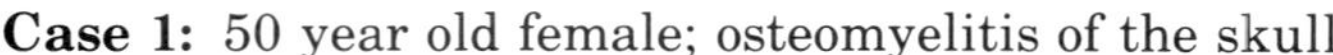

Case 1: 50 year old female; osteomyelitis of the skull

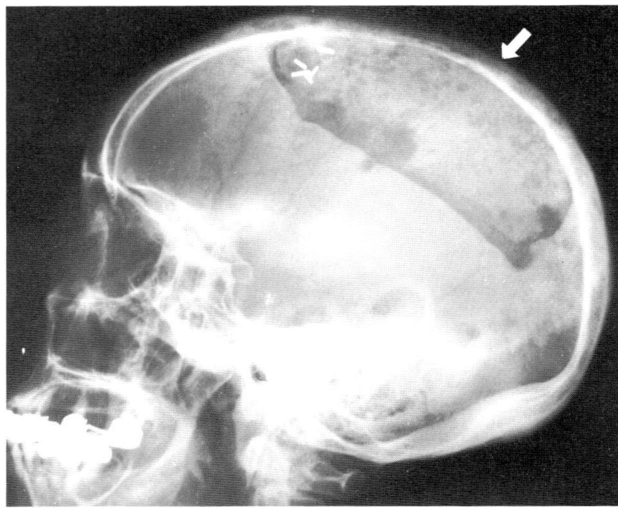

Fig. 15

A parasagittal meningioma had been removed a year before the present examination. For the immediate past two weeks, a persistent high temperature was present. A cutaneous fistula with pus drainage was seen on the skin. An X-ray revealed a worm-eaten appearance of the post-operative bone flap, typical of osteomyelitis.

Case 2: 28 year old male; pituitary adenoma

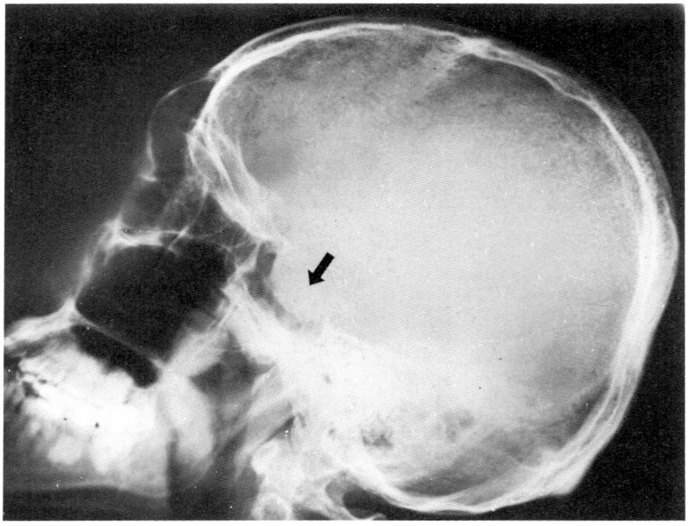

Fig. 16

Chief complaint was impairment of vision. After hospitalization, neurological examination revealed a bitemporal hemianopia. X-ray showed an expansion of the sella turcica, the so-called "ballooning effect" (←). The tumor, subsequently removed through the nasal cavity, was found to be a prolactinoma (a type of pituitary adenoma).

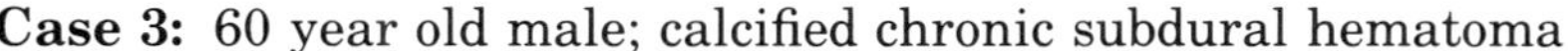

Case 3: 60 year old male; calcified chronic subdural hematoma

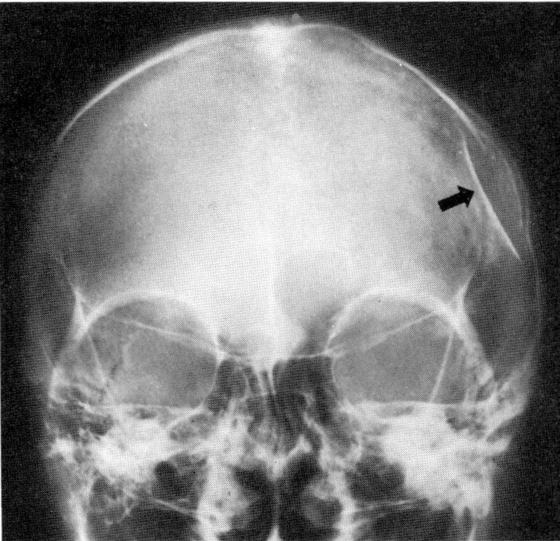

Fig. 17

Headache had been repeatedly evident for ten years, becoming more intense immediately before the patient's visit. On first examination, no specific neurological abnormality was detected. X-ray revealed a membranous calcified shadow (→), concave medially, in the upper part of the right temporal bone. This may have had no bearing on the patient's headache. Rather, it was suggestive of chronic subdural hematoma which had calcified without ill effect and without the patient's knowledge.

Case 4: 21 year old male; skull fracture (acute extradural hematoma)

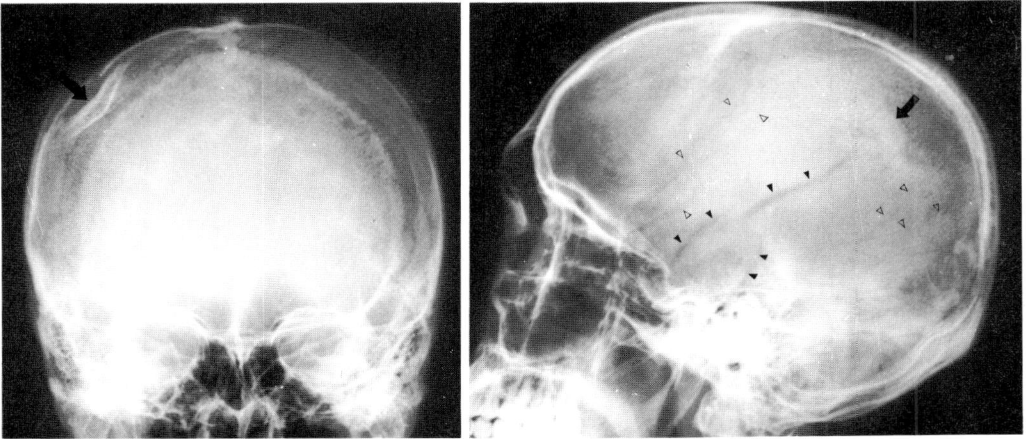

Fig. 18

The patient was hit by a car while riding a bicycle. His senses became muddled while receiving first aid for an injury to the left parietal region. Four hours later, he was examined for neurological signs. With impaired awareness, he exhibited little response to pain. An anteroposterior projection X-ray revealed little damage except for a depressed fracture in the left parietal region (→). In the lateral plane, the depression was not obvious, but a few associated linear fractures were detected (▶). Note the difference in appearance between these fractures and various blood vessel grooves (▷).

MENINGEAL COVERINGS OF THE BRAIN

The brain is protected by a series of three membranous coverings: the outermost dura mater (6–8), the arachnoid (6–9), and the innermost pia mater.

The innermost pia mater is the thinnest of these membranes. It closely invests the brain's surface, following all the contours of its sulci.

The arachnoid membrane is also thin. It's association is less intimate with the brain, skipping over the sulci. Between the arachnoid and the pia, there are small strands of arachnoid tissue, shaped like a spider's web (= Greek, arachne). The space under the arachnoid is called the subarachnoid space (6–10), in which cerebrospinal fluid flows and subarachnoidal hemorrhage can occur.

The outermost dura mater completely covers the inner surface of the cranium. The dura is actually composed of two membranes, the outer periosteum and the true inner dura mater. These are clinically indistinguishable except for some spaces between it and the outer periosteum (which provide venous drainage), the dural sinuses (6–15, 19–1, 3, 6, 7).

The dura mater has two important reflections within the cranium. One, called the falx cerebri (= Latin, sickle), is a sagittal reflection, shaped like a grass-cutting sickle (6–16, 19–2, 20–1). The falx helps separate the two cerebral hemispheres. Learning the position and shape of the falx is important for understanding the falx sign, which is evident occasionally on an angiogram.

Another key reflection is called the tentorium cerebelli (19–5, 20–2). It forms two plates of the tentorial pyramid. Another plate, called the incisura tentorii or tentorial hiatus (19–A), allows passage of the midbrain. The tentorium cerebelli is contacted on its upper surface by the temporal and the occipital lobes, and by the cerebellum on its under surface. Recognition of the incisura tentorii is important for understanding a tentorial herniation, as described later.

The terms supratentorial and infratentorial are important for distinguishing between damage on either side of the tentorium cerebelli (Fig. 19). They represent quite different clinical signs and plans of treatment.

Some sensory branches of the trigeminal nerve are distributed to the dura mater and the arachnoid. Their sensory input serves the recognition of headache. There are no pain receptors in the brain's substance. This was known even in ancient times, when brain surgery was often performed under local or no anesthesia. Thus, headache is attributable to noxious sensory input from the meningeal membranes. In cases of increasing intracranial pressure, intracranial hemorrhage (especially, subarachnoid hemorrhage) or inflammation, the sensory endings of trigeminal axons are activated, leading to the perception of headache. The combination of this headache with a stiff neck (Nackenstarre) and positive Kernig sign* is an important clinical sign of meningeal irritation.

---

*Positive Kernig sign: With the patient in the supine position with flexed knees, a thigh is raised perpendicular to the ground. The knee is then extended passively. Full extension is usually possible in normal subjects. However, in patients with meningeal irritation, the knee cannot be extended fully because of pain or reflex twitching.

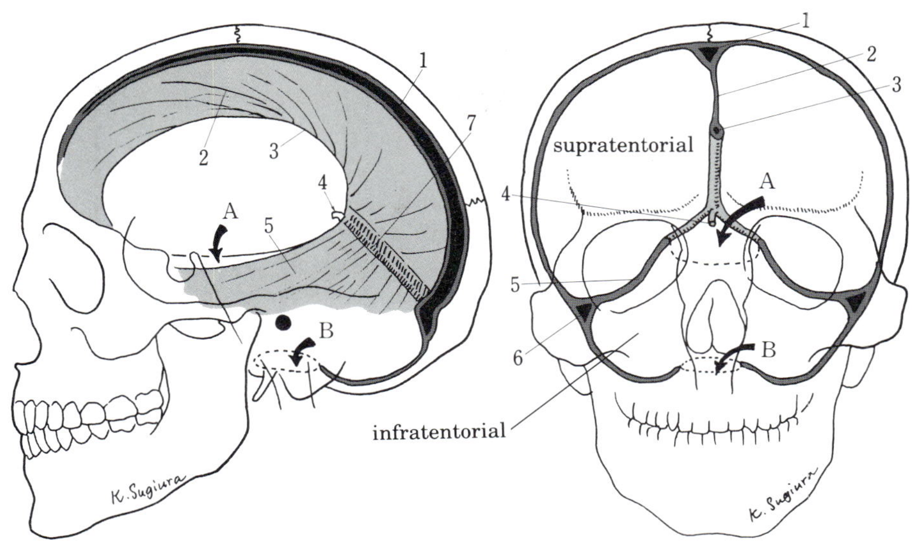

Fig. 19 The dura mater and sinus.

1. superior sagittal sinus
2. falx cerebri
3. inferior sagittal sinus
4. great cerebral vein
5. tentorium cerebelli
6. transverse sinus
7. straight sinus

A. tentorial incisura
B. foramen magnum

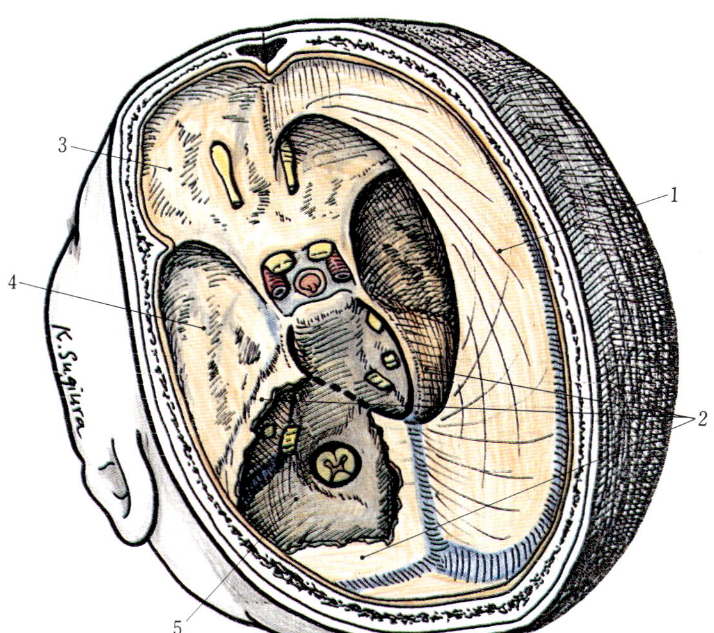

1. falx cerebri
2. tentorium cerebelli
3. anterior cranial fossa
4. middle cranial fossa
5. posterior cranial fossa

Fig. 20 The falx cerebri and tentorium cerebelli.
The posterior cranial fossa is shown by removal of the tentorium cerebelli.

3. THE VASCULAR SYSTEM

ARTERIES

The brain is supplied by four arteries, a pair of internal carotid arteries and a pair of vertebral arteries.

The internal carotid artery (21, 22–1) passes through the cranial base (petrous part of the temporal bone) to enter the cranium and advances into the cavernous sinus forming part of the carotid siphon (21–2). It then penetrates the dura mater to finally enter the cranial space (in the neurosurgical sense). Posteriorly it connects with the posterior communicating artery and terminates at the branching point of the anterior cerebral artery and the middle cerebral artery.

The anterior cerebral artery proceeds antero-medially over the optic nerve (22–6) and enters the cerebral fissure between the left and right hemispheres. Next, it turns upward and posteriorly to approach the corpus callosum in the median plane (Fig. 63). Here, it bifurcates into progressively smaller branches, and finally terminates. Since the anterior cerebral artery normally courses in the median plane, its deviation to the left or right of this plane in an antero-posterior view of an angiogram (so-called "shift") has special significance. The left and the right anterior cerebral arteries are connected by the anterior communicating artery (22–7), located directly above the optic chiasma. This artery is a frequent site for aneurysms.

The large middle cerebral artery (21, 22–5) proceeds laterally and horizontally for about 3 cm, deep in the fissure of Sylvius, where it divides into many branches. These branches, also called the Sylvian group (Fig. 32, 33), run on the surface of the triangle-shaped insula of Reil before proceeding to their distribution areas (Fig. 59, 60). Displacement of these arterial branches from the normal triangle, as observed in a lateral angiogram of the carotid artery, can be used to detect the location of a tumor.

The left and right vertebral arteries (21, 22–8) enter the cranial space through the foramen magnum (10–24, 19–B). They proceed supero-medially, with branches forming the posterior inferior cerebellar arteries (PICA) (22–9). These meet at the midline to form the single basilar artery (21, 22–10) which proceeds supero-anteriorly over the pons and gives off branches called the anterior inferior cerebellar artery (AICA) (22–11) and the superior cerebellar artery (22–12). The basilar artery finally ends at the branching point of left and right posterior cerebral arteries (21, 22–13), which run along the tentorium on the incisura margin. They connect with the internal carotid arteries by way of a branch called the posterior communicating artery. The posterior cerebral arteries continue around the cerebral peduncle, turn posteriorly and proceed close to the medio-inferior surface of the temporal lobe to finally terminate within each occipital lobe.

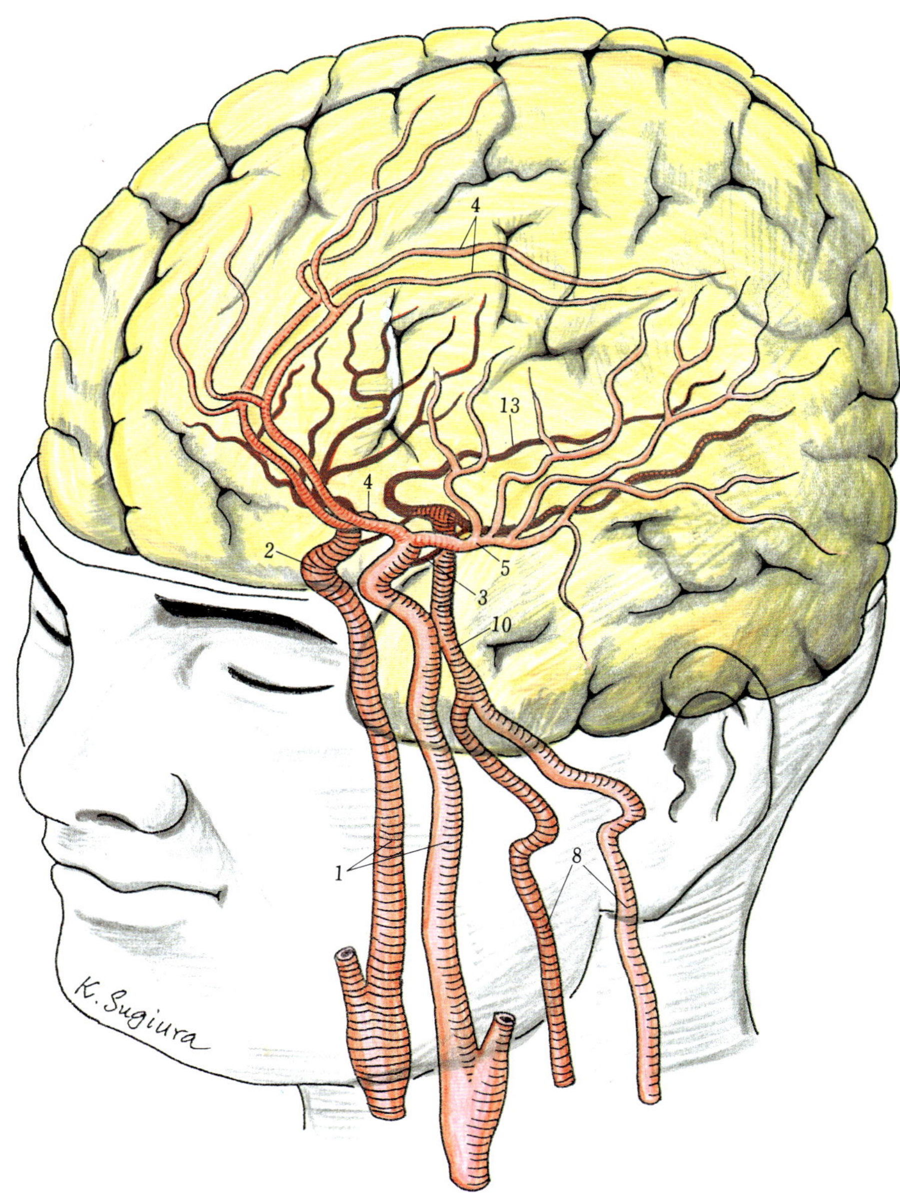

Fig. 21 Arteries of the brain.

1. internal carotid artery
2. carotid siphon
3. posterior communicating artery
4. anterior cerebral artery
5. middle cerebral artery
(6. chiasma)
(7. anterior communicating artery)
8. vertebral artery
(9. posterior-inferior cerebellar artery)
10. basilar artery
(11. anterior-inferior cerebellar artery)
(12. superior cerebellar artery)
13. posterior cerebral artery
(14. infundibulum of hypophysis)
(15. anterior choroidal artery)
(16. posterior choroidal artery)

Note: Structure in parentheses is shown in Figure 22.

CIRCLE OF WILLIS: The anterior cerebral arteries (22–4) connect by way of an anterior communicating artery (22–7). Similarly, each posterior cerebral artery is connected to the internal carotid artery (22–1) by a posterior communicating artery (22–3). This completes an arterial loop, called the circle of Willis, around the optic nerve (22–6) and the infundibular stalk (22–14). It serves an important role for anastomotic flow. Cerebral aneurysms mostly occur within the circle, causing subarachnoid hemorrhage. The large arteries shown in Fig. 21, 22 all course within the subarachnoid space. They divide into progressively smaller arteries and arterioles, before entering the brain's substance where they terminate as capillaries.

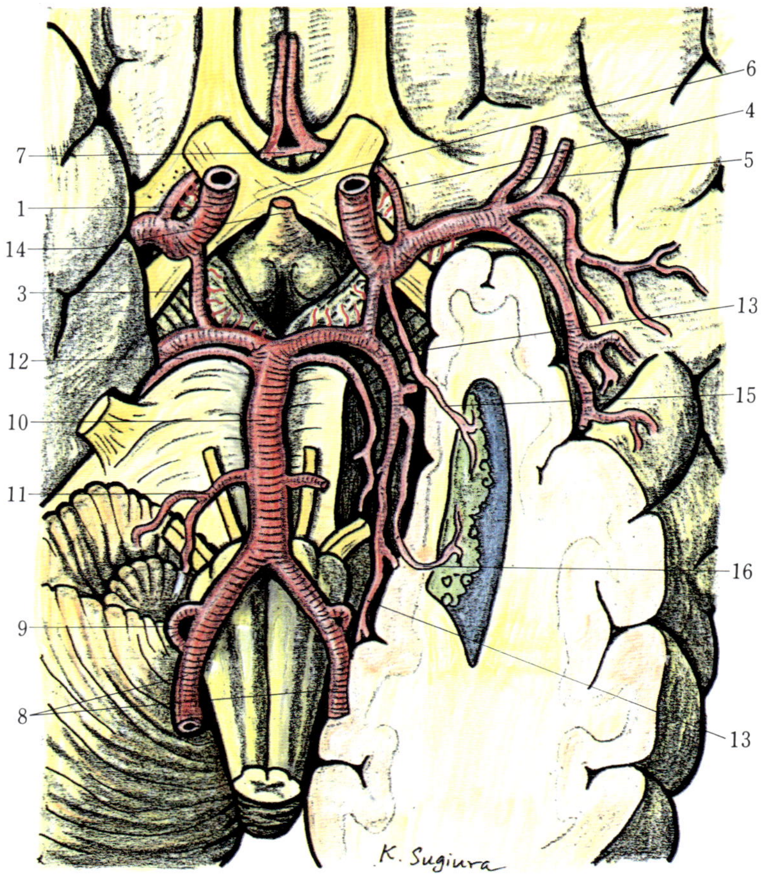

Fig. 22 The cerebral arterial circle (of Willis).

1. internal carotid artery
(2. carotid siphon)
3. posterior communicating artery
4. anterior cerebral artery
5. middle cerebral artery
6. chiasma
7. anterior communicating artery
8. vertebral artery
9. posterior-inferior cerebellar artery
10. basilar artery
11. anterior-inferior cerebellar artery
12. superior cerebellar artery
13. posterior cerebral artery
14. infundibulum of hypophysis
15. anterior choroidal artery
16. posterior choroidal artery

Note: Structure in parentheses is shown in Figure 21.

VEINS

Venous systems around the brain stem and under the tentorium are not covered in this text but Fig. 23 provides an overall understanding. The venous drainage of the cerebrum is brought about by three systems: superficial cerebral veins (23–1, 2), deep cerebral veins (23–3 ~ 10) and the anastomotic veins of Trolard (23–11) and Labbe (23–12) which connect the former two systems. The larger veins course in passages formed in the dura mater. Here, they are called venous sinuses.

Among the dural sinuses shown in Fig. 23, the superior sagittal, transverse and sigmoid sinuses are important for understanding traumatic injury. If these dural sinuses are injured by the edge of a cranial fracture, a hematoma forms in the sub- or extra-dural space. Thalamostriate veins and the great cerebral vein of Galen should especially be noted among the deep cerebral veins. The former courses along the outer wall of the body of the lateral ventricle, which helps when examining for hydrocephalus. The great cerebral vein is clinically important due to its several anatomical anomalies and to pinealoma.

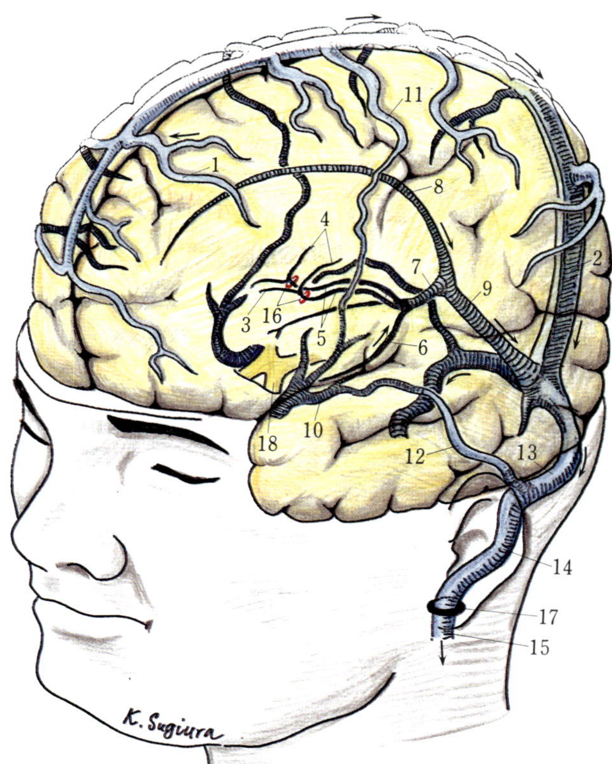

Fig. 23 Veins of the brain

1. superficial cerebral veins
2. superior sagittal sinus
3. septal vein
4. thalamostriate vein
5. internal cerebral vein
6. basal vein (of Rosenthal)
7. great cerebral vein (of Galen)
8. inferior sagittal sinus
9. straight sinus
10. superficial middle cerebral vein
11. superior anastomotic vein (of Trolard)
12. inferior anastomotic vein (of Labbe)
13. transverse sinus
14. sigmoid sinus
15. internal jugular vein
16. foramina of Monro
17. jugular foramen
18. optic nerve

ARTERIAL SUPPLY OF THE BRAIN

Figures 24 , 25 show areas supplied by the cerebral arteries. The anterior, middle and posterior cerebral arteries mainly supply the medio-frontal, lateral and posterior-inferior surfaces of the brain, respectively. Recognition of these distributions aids in locating the artery responsible for a cerebral infarct, as revealed by computerized tomography, which is explained below. It should also be noted that while the anterior choroidal artery and arterial ramifications from the circle of Willis have small diameters, they nonetheless play an important role in supplying the internal capsule and thalamus, deep in the center of the brain (Fig. 25).

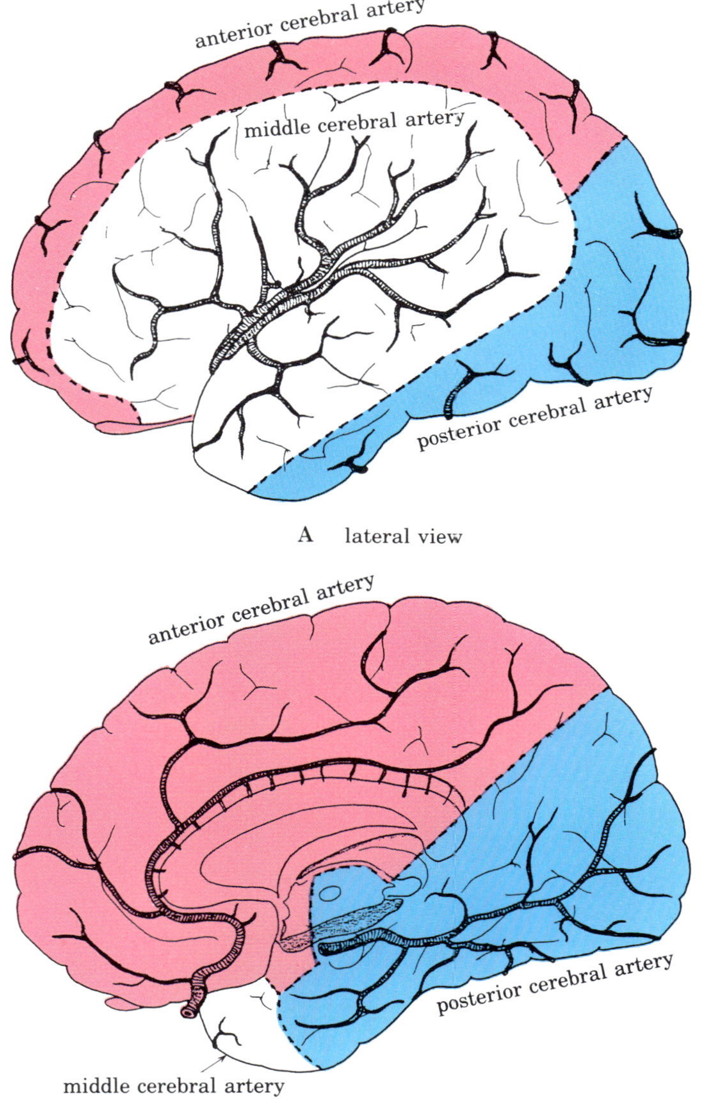

Fig. 24 Distribution of arteries to the cerebral cortex (after Chusid).

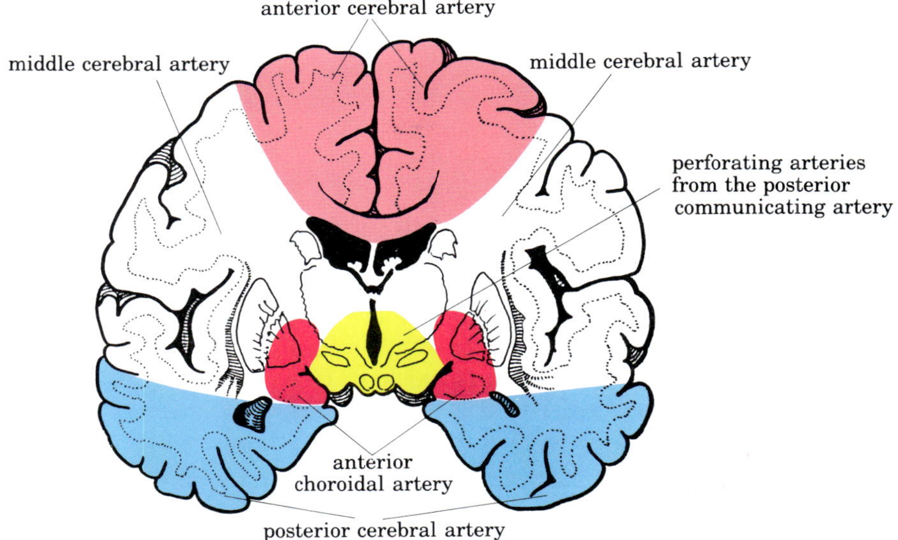

A coronal section

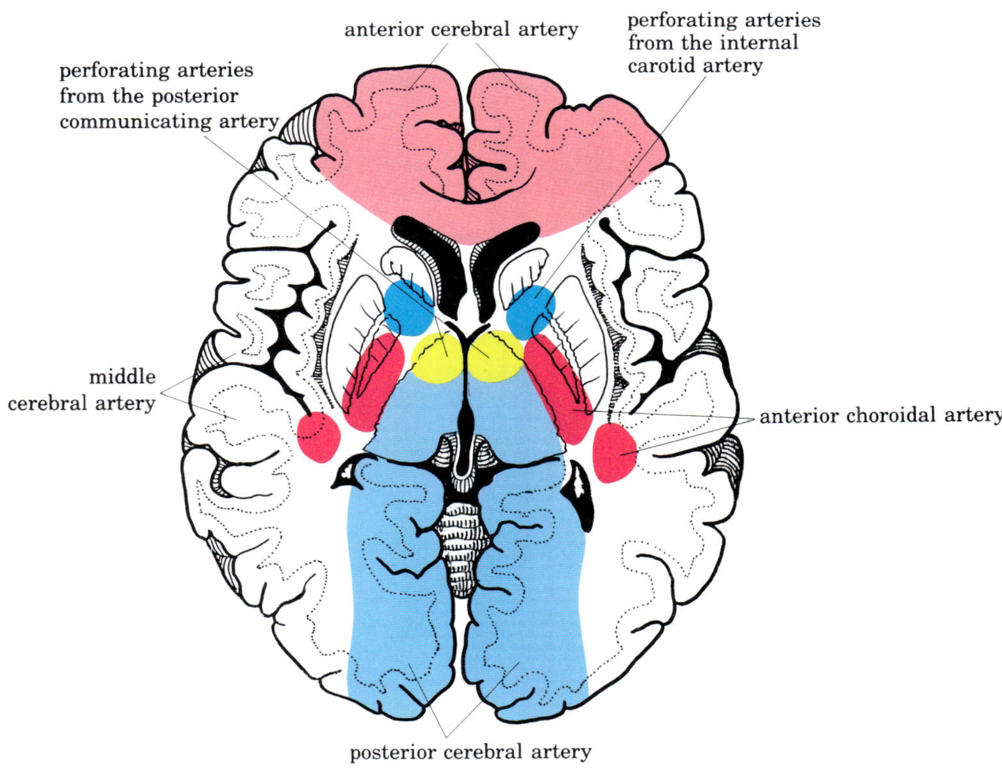

B horizontal section

Fig. 25 The brain's arterial supply shown in sections (after Chusid).

CEREBRAL ANGIOGRAPHY

Angiography is the most important examination technique yet devised for diagnosing blood-vessel diseases such as cerebral aneurysms and arterio-venous anomalies. It reveals blood vessels of the brain by means of X-ray, after injection of contrast media into a carotid or vertebral artery.

Angiography started with the 1920's work of Egas Moniz (a Portuguese neurosurgeon). Initially, he had little success with percutaneous injection of contrast media, but was more successful when injections were made directly into an artery exposed in the neck. The later development of percutaneous angiography was greatly aided by Japanese workers, including Shimizu and Sano.

Cerebral angiography was developed after pneumography (1919), but it quickly became the more reliable neurosurgical tool. However, the role of angiography is now gradually diminishing, having been replaced in many instances by computerized tomography (CT, as described later), a safer procedure that also provides more information.

Knowledge of anatomy is essential for the examination of angiograms of both the carotid and vertebral arteries. Figures 26–37 provide examples of normal angiograms.

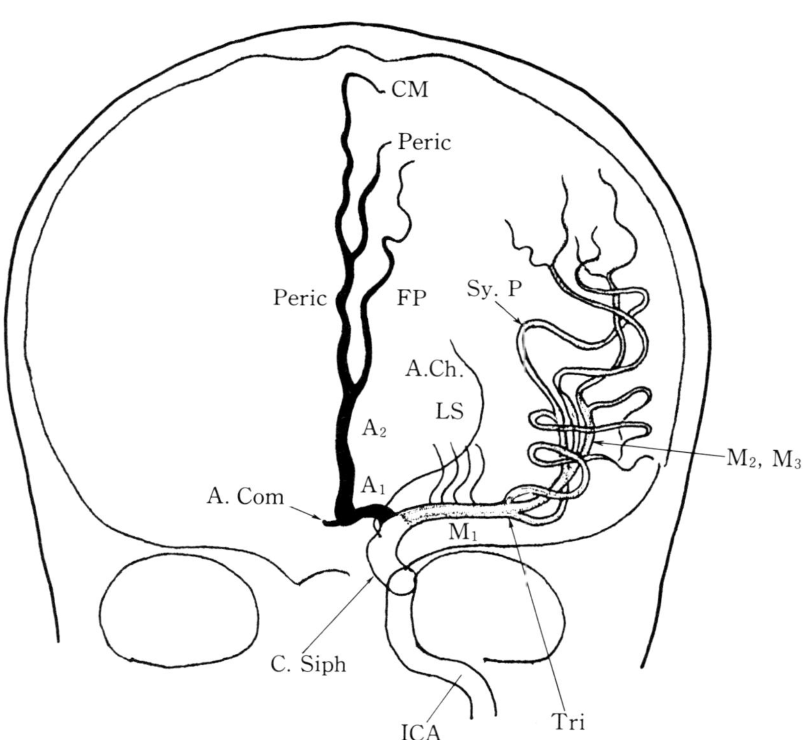

Fig. 26 A diagram drawn from an angiogram of a normal carotid artery; antero-posterior view.

A1, A2, A3: segments of the anterior cerebral artery (a.)
A.Ch.: anterior choroidal a.
A.Com.: anterior communicating a.
CM: callosomarginal a.
C. Siph.: carotid siphon
FP: frontopolar a.
ICA: internal carotid a.
LS: lenticulostriate a.
M1, M2, M3: segments of the middle cerebral a.
Oph: ophthalmic a.
PC: posterior cerebral a.
P.Com.: posterior communicating a.
Peric: pericallosal a.
Sy.P.: Sylvian point

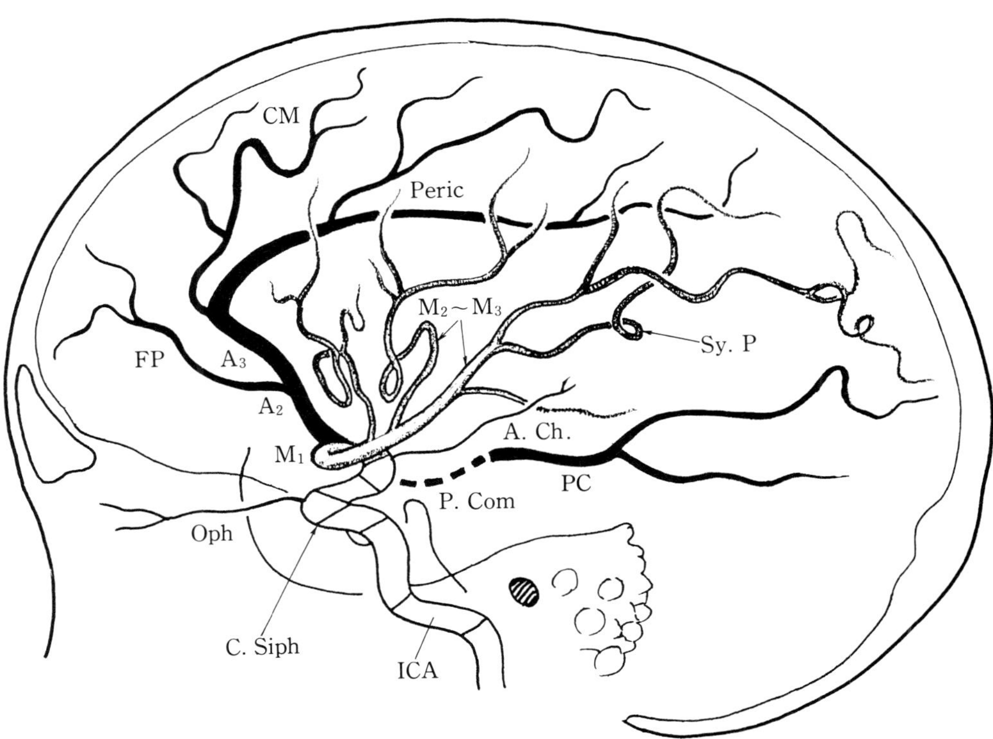

Fig. 27 A diagram from an angiogram of a normal carotid artery; lateral view.

BVR: basilar vein of Rosenthal
C: cavernous sinus
ICV: internal cerebral vein
IS: inferior sagittal sinus
MCV: middle cerebral vein
O: occipital sinus
Sig: sigmoid sinus
SP: superior petrosal sinus

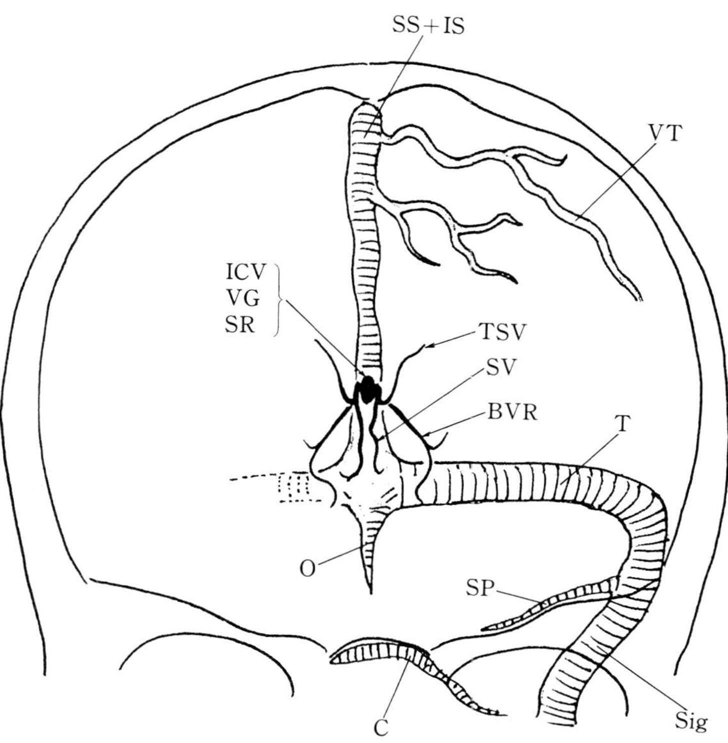

Fig. 28 A diagram from an angiogram of a normal carotid artery, showing parts of the venous system; antero-posterior view.

SR: sinus rectus
SS: superior sagittal sinus
SV: septal vein
T: transverse sinus
TSV: thalamostriate vein
VA: venous angle
VG: vein of Galen
VL: vein of Labbe
VT: vein of Trolard

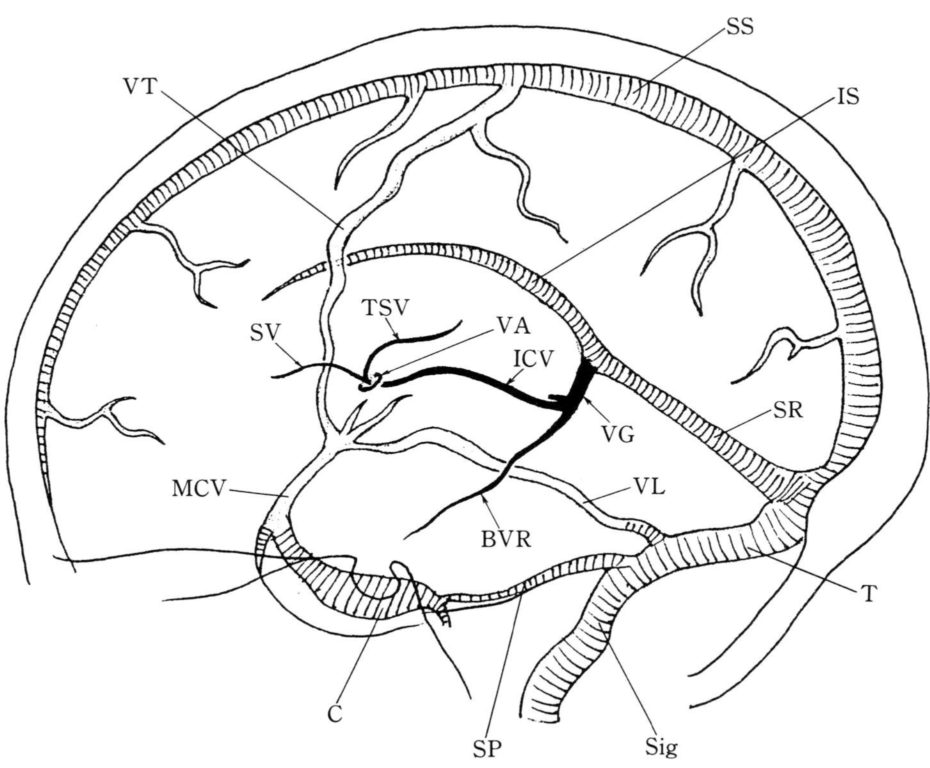

Fig. 29 A diagram from an angiogram of a normal carotid artery, showing parts of the venous system; lateral view.

AICA: anterior inferior cerebellar a.
BA: basilar a.
BT: basilar top
DCC: dorsal a. of the corpus callosum
PC: posterior cerebral a.
P. Ch.: posterior choroidal a.
P. Com.: posterior communicating a.

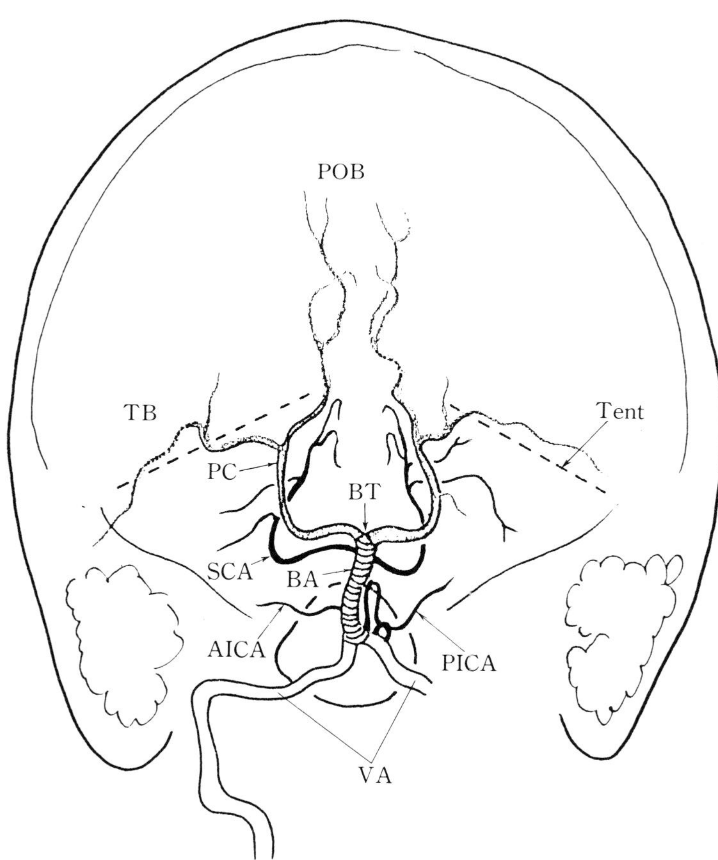

Fig. 30 A diagram from an angiogram of a normal vertebral artery; antero-posterior view.

PICA: posterior inferior cerebellar a.
POB: parieto-occipital branch of the posterior cerebral a.
P. Th.: posterior thalamoperforating a.
SCA: superior cerebellar a.
TB: temporal branch of the posterior cerebral a.
Tent: tentorium cerebelli
VA: vertebral a.

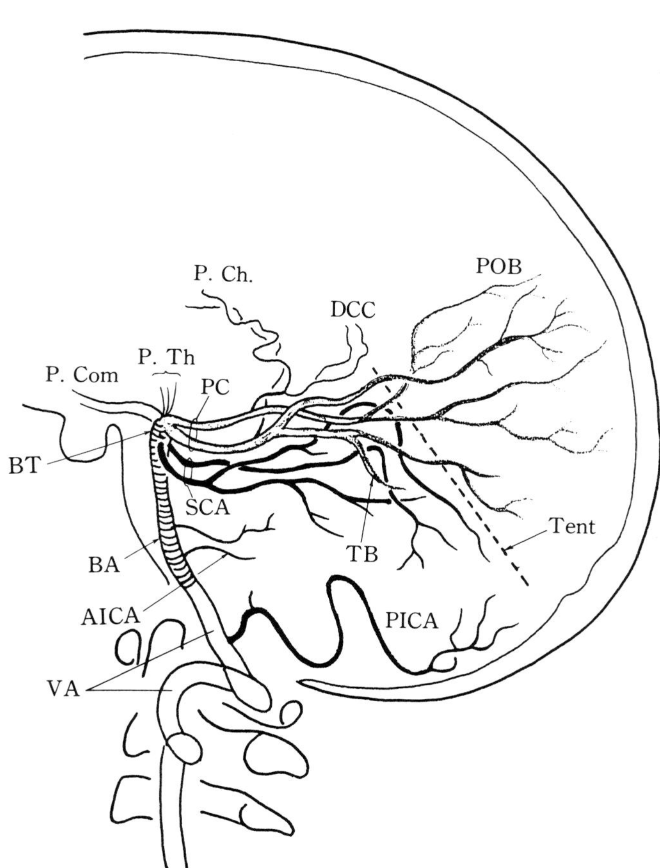

Fig. 31 A diagram from an angiogram of a normal vertebral artery; lateral view.

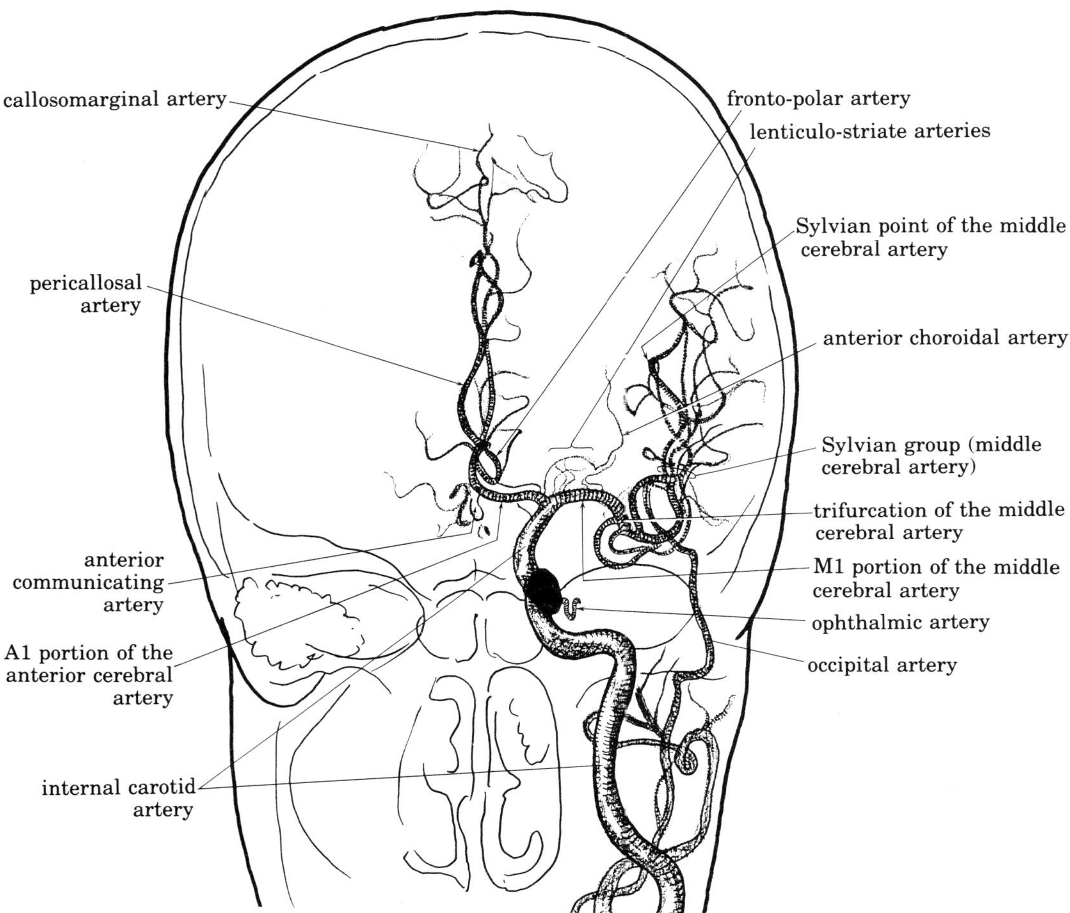

Fig. 32A A diagram from an angiogram of a normal carotid artery; frontal view (Drawn from Fig. 32B; same subject as in Fig. 33.)

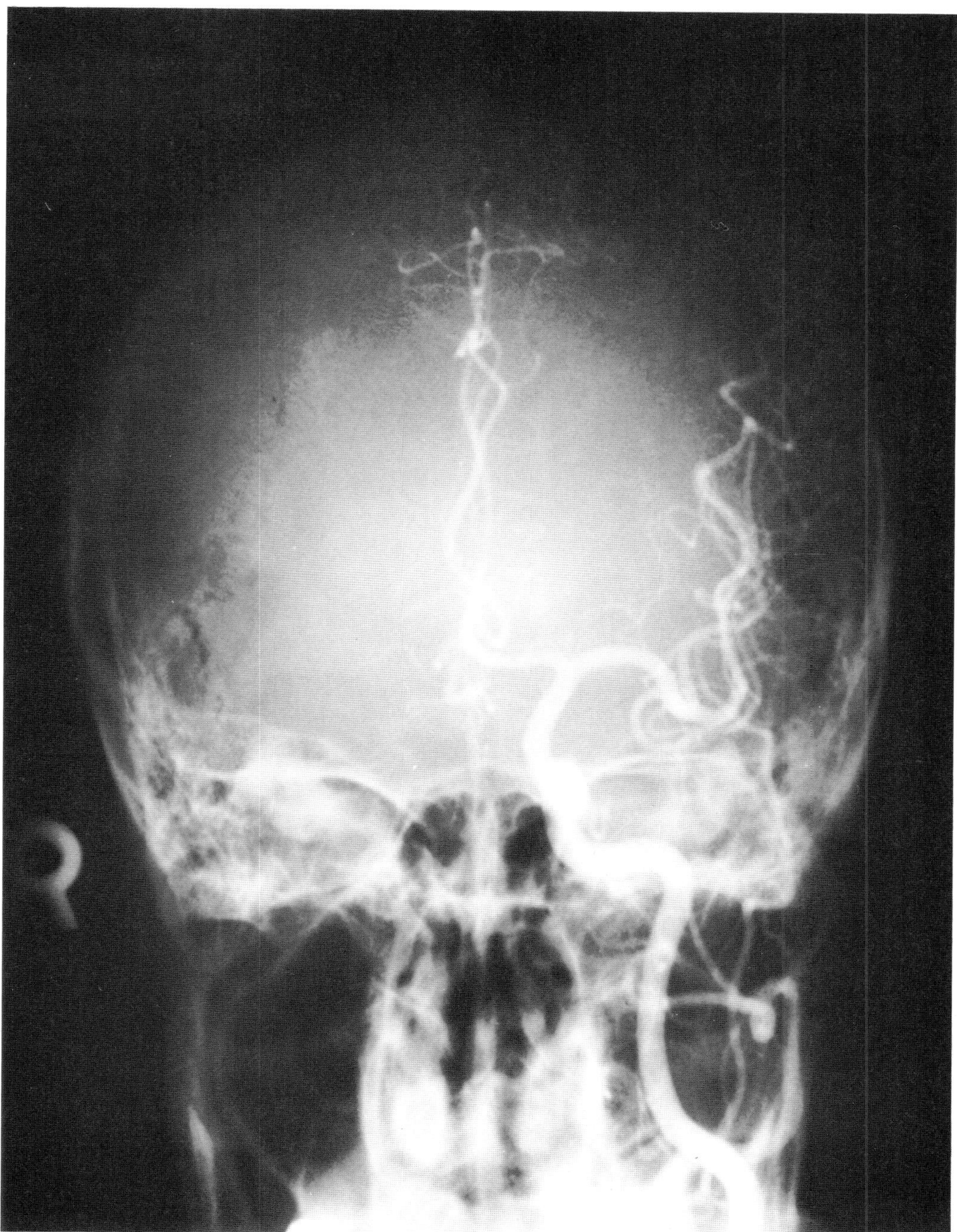

Fig. 32B An angiogram of a normal carotid artery; frontal view

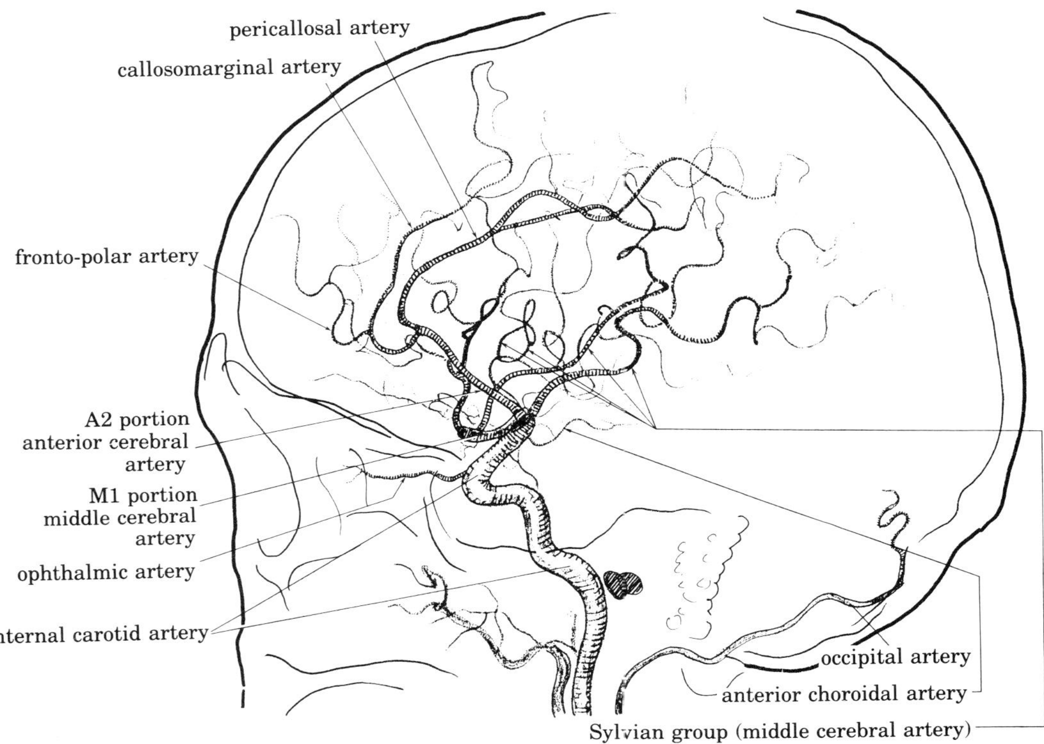

Fig. 33A A diagram of an angiogram of a normal carotid artery; lateral view.

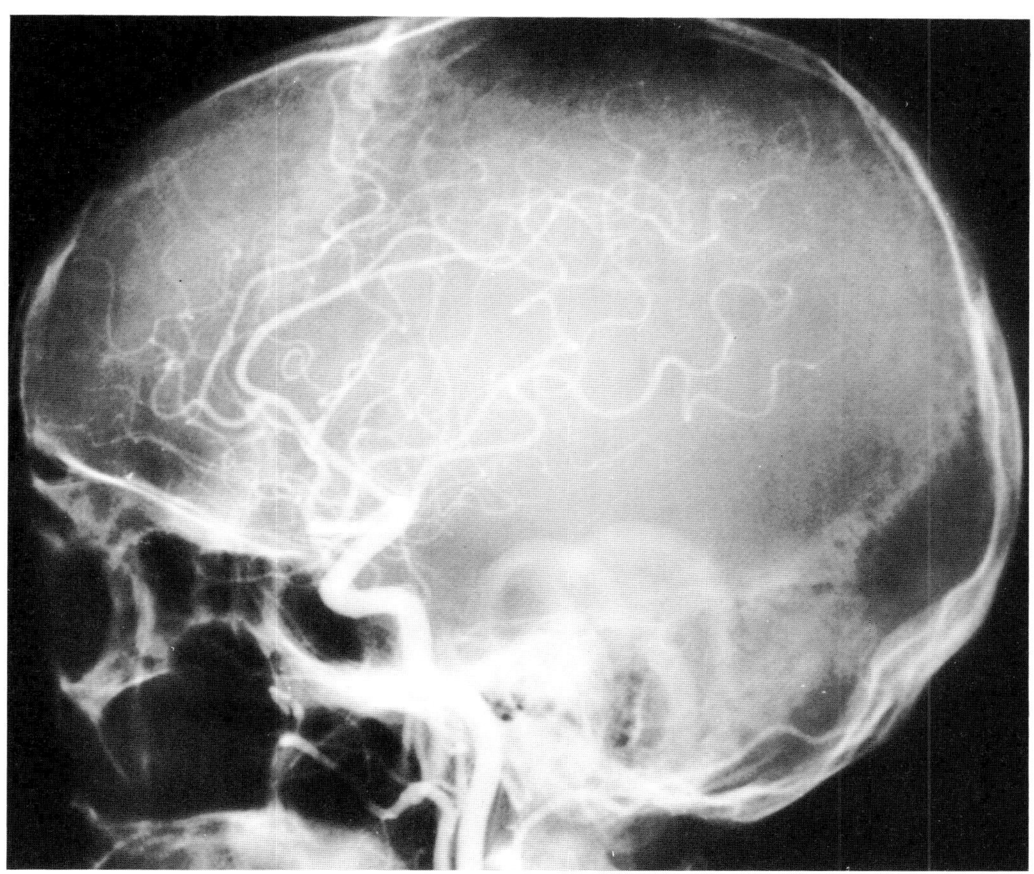

Fig. 33B An angiogram of a normal carotid artery; lateral view.

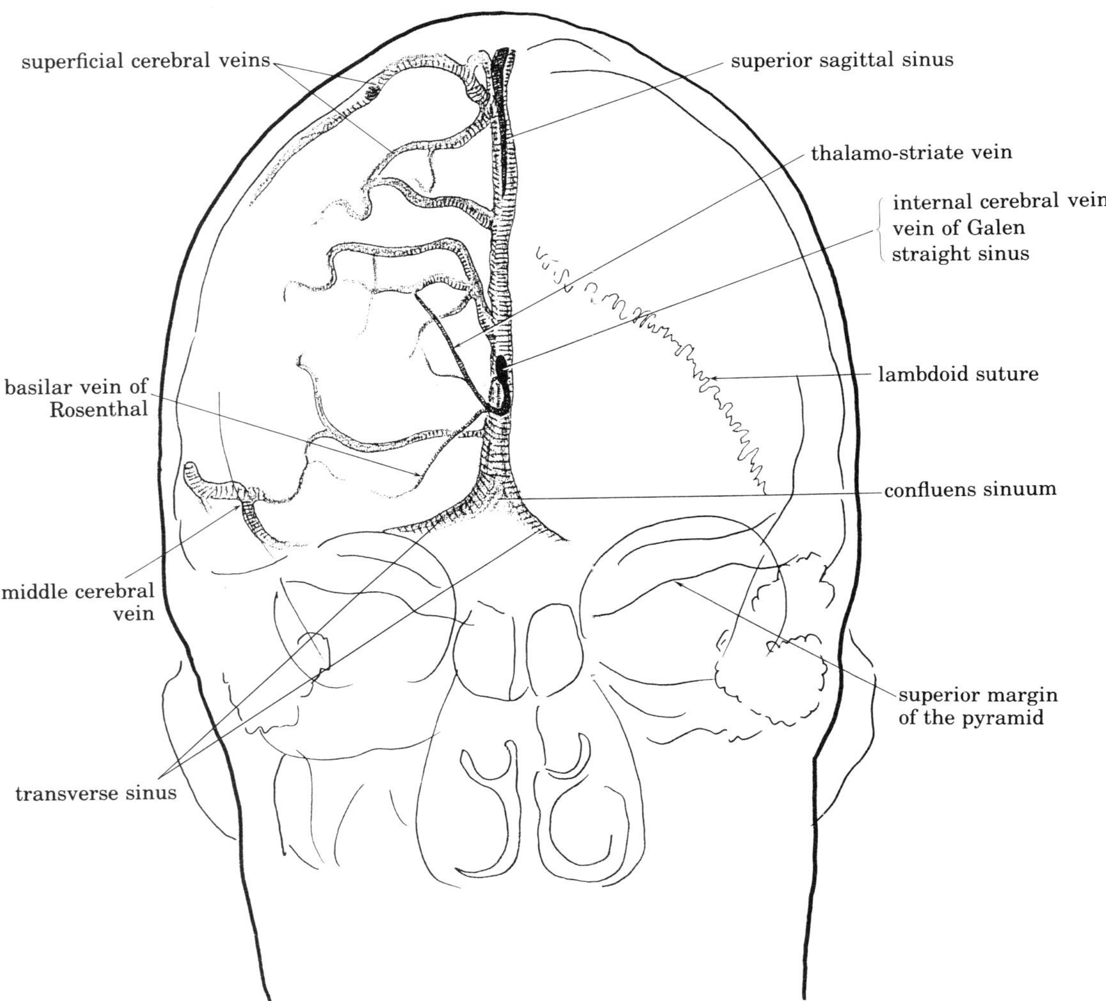

Fig. 34A A diagram from an angiogram of the normal carotid artery showing parts of the venous system; frontal view (Drawn from Fig. 34B; same subject in Fig. 35).

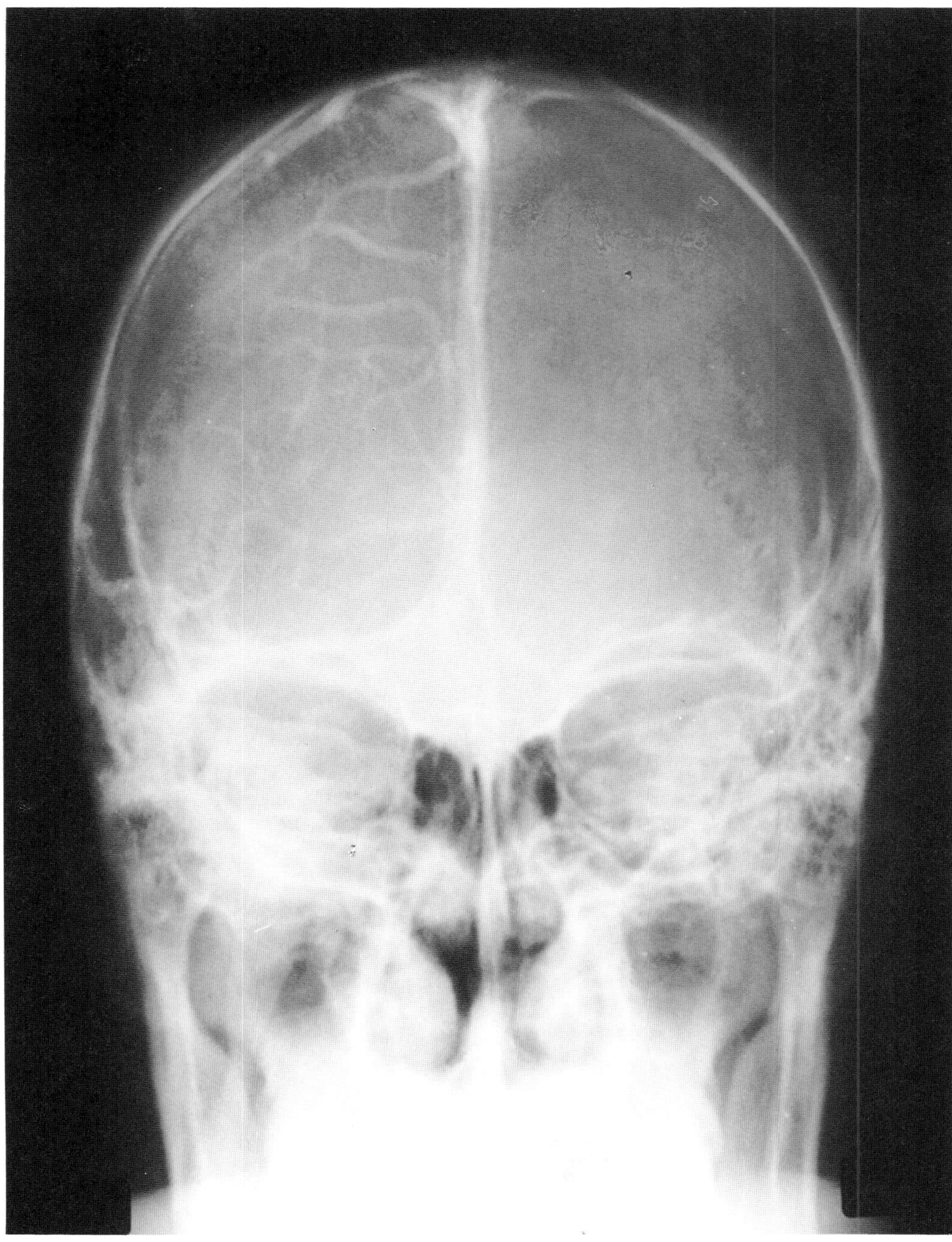

Fig. 34B An angiogram of a normal carotid artery showing parts of the venous system; frontal view.

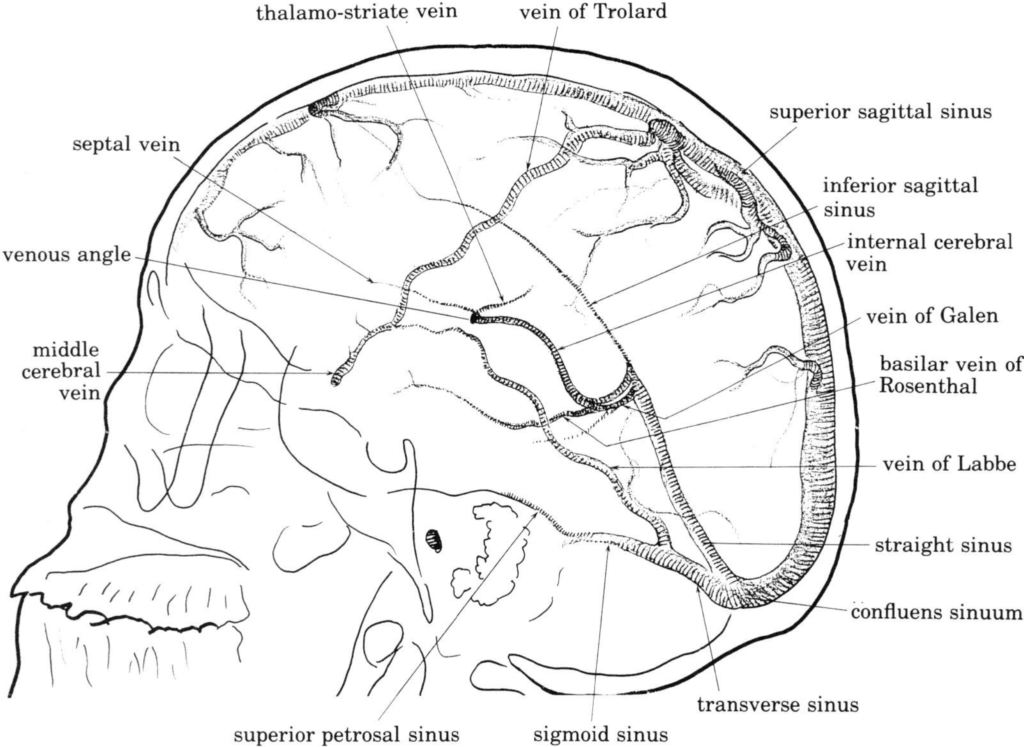

Fig. 35A A diagram from an angiogram of the normal carotid artery showing parts of the venous system; lateral view (Drawn from Fig. 35B).

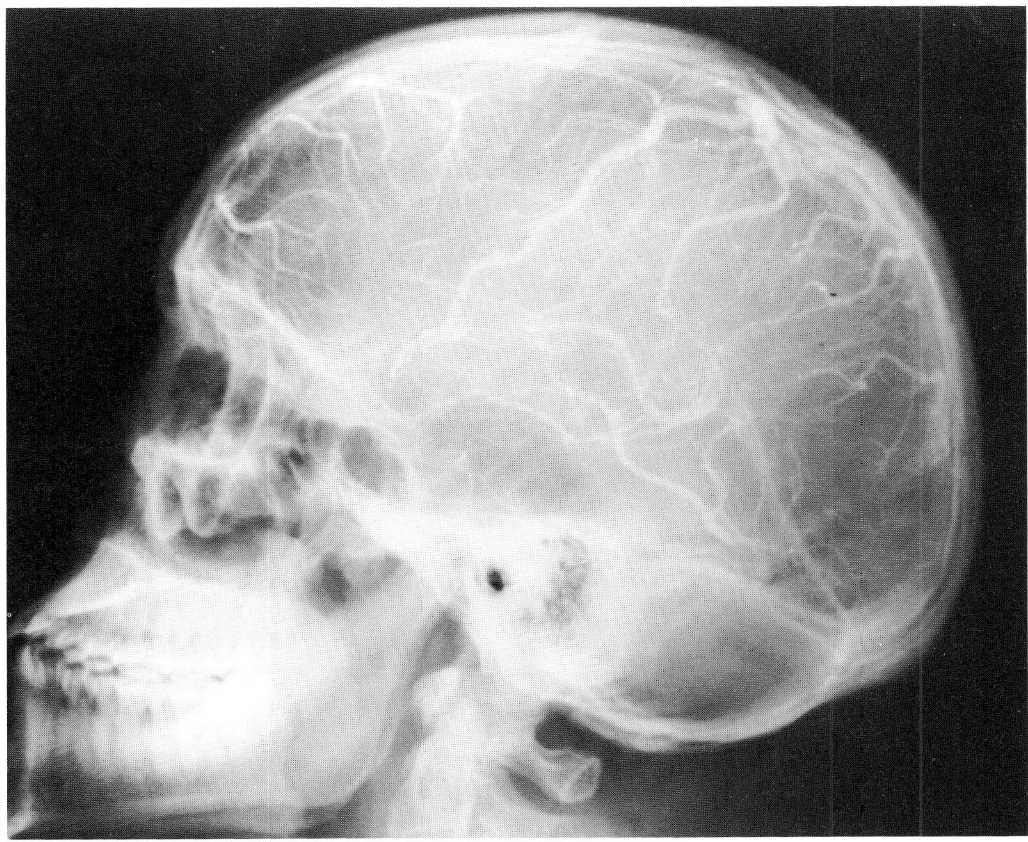

Fig. 35B An angiogram of a normal carotid artery showing parts of the venous system; lateral view.

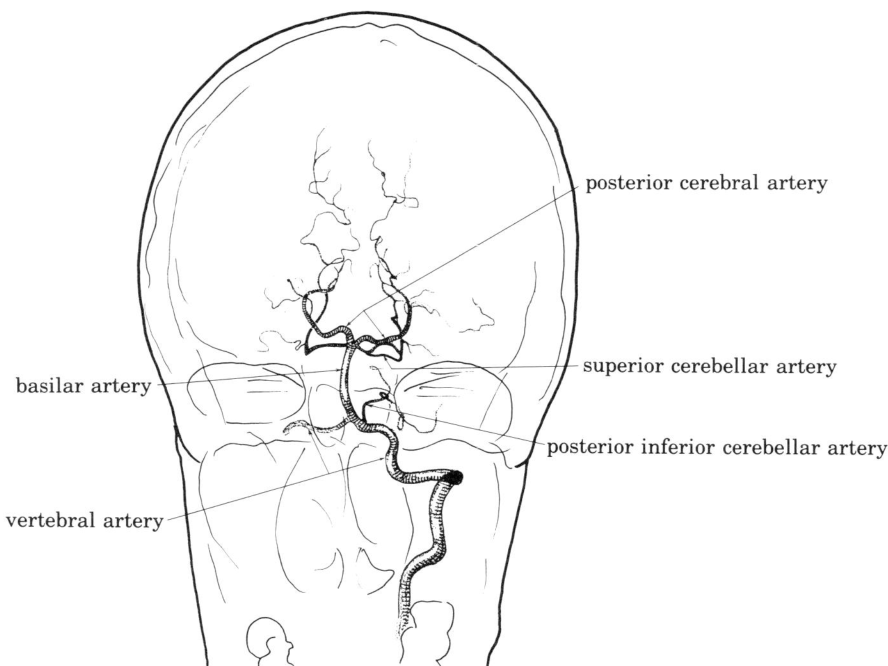

Fig. 36A A diagram of an angiogram of a normal vertebral artery; frontal view (Drawn from Fig. 36B).

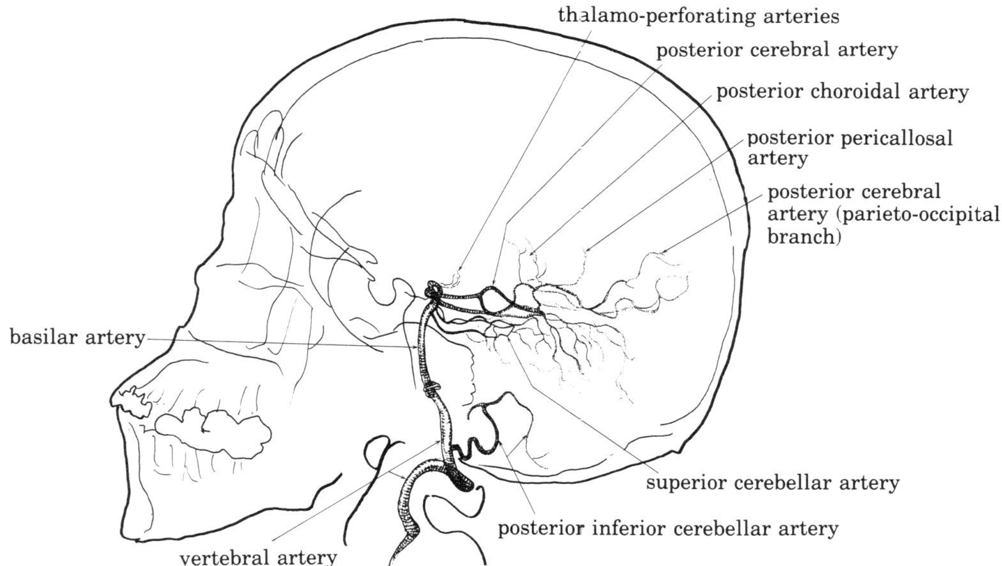

Fig. 37A A diagram of an angiogram of a normal vertebral artery; lateral view (Drawn from Fig. 37B).

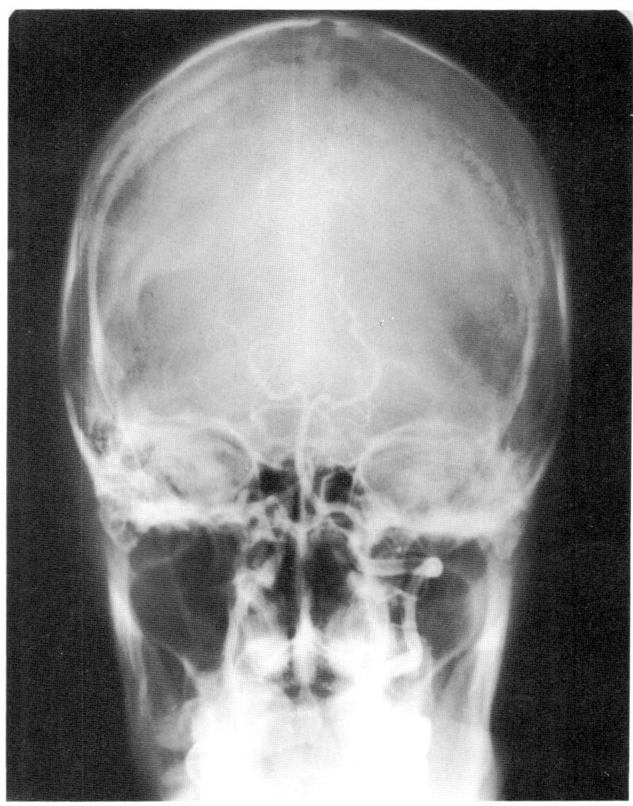

Fig. 36B An angiogram of a normal vertebral artery; frontal view.

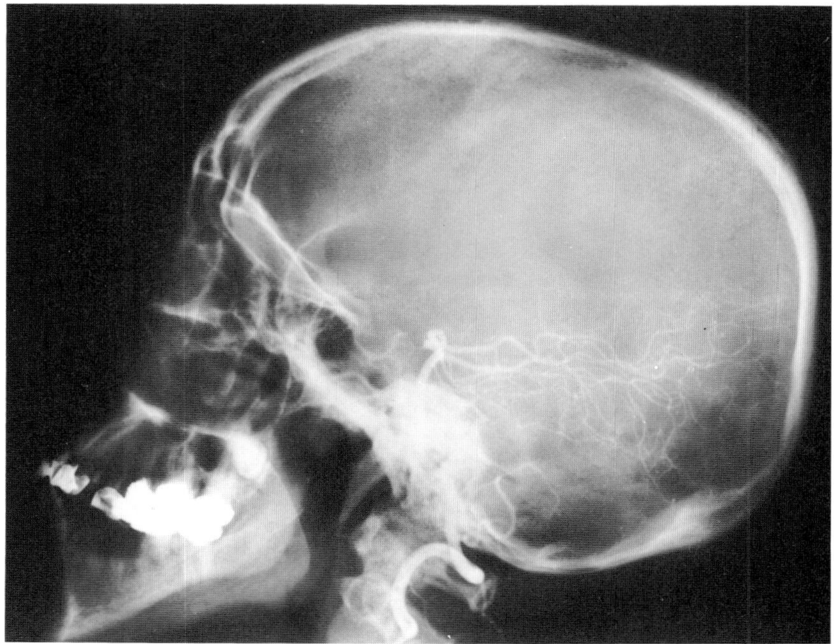

Fig. 37B An angiogram of a normal vertebral artery; lateral view.

Case 5: 36 year old male; occlusion of the middle cerebral artery 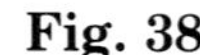 **Fig. 38**

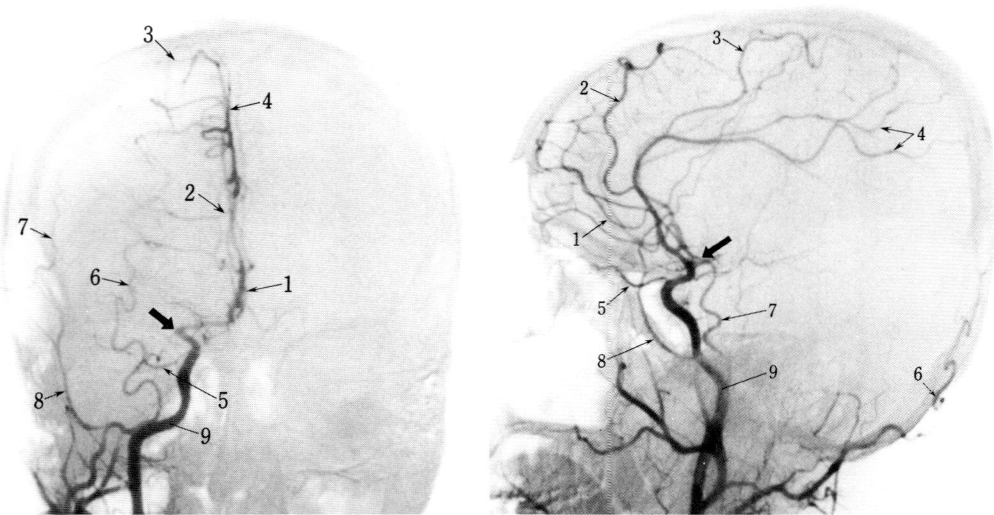

Patient felt dizzy while walking, and then fell down. When hospitalized, he was conscious, but had a speech disorder and left side paralysis of the body. Heart disease was noted on his clinical record, and a mitral valve lesion was suspected from auscultation of the heart. The middle cerebral artery was not seen beyond its point of origin (Fig. 38, →). Instead, branches of the anterior cerebral and external carotid arteries were conspicuous. An embolus from the heart may have blocked the right middle cerebral artery. 1) frontobasal a; 2) frontopolar a; 3) posterior medial frontal a; 4) medial parietal branch of callosomarginal a; 5) ophthalmic a; 6) occipital a; 7) superficial temporal a; 8) middle meningeal a; 9) internal carotid a.

Case 6: 67 year old female; malignant astrocytoma **Fig. 39**

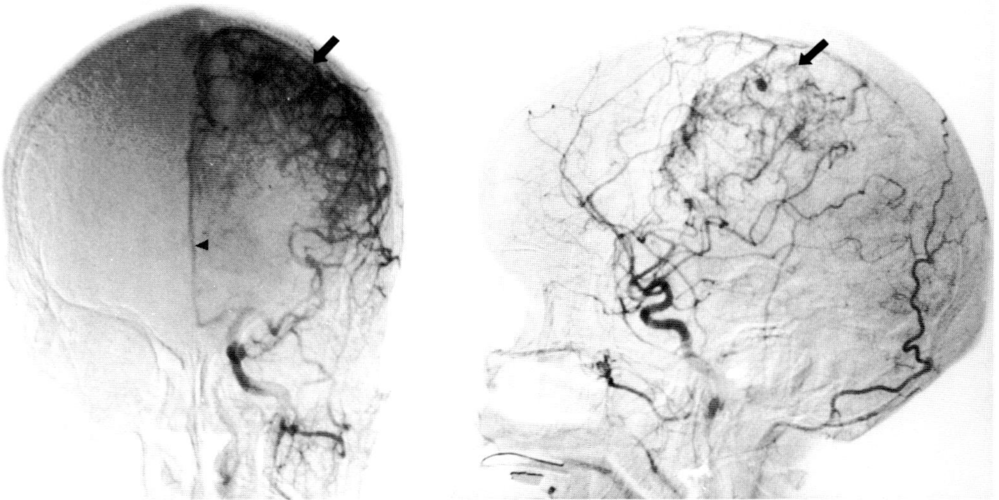

Chief complaints were aphasia and right half paralysis of the body which gradually became more severe during the 7 months prior to examination. Abnormal and irregular blood vessels in the parietal region are evident (→), but displacement of the anterior cerebral artery (◀) is slight. Pathological diagnosis of the removed tissue was malignant astrocytoma.

Case 7: 30 year old male; arterio-venous malformation **Fig. 40**

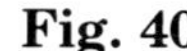

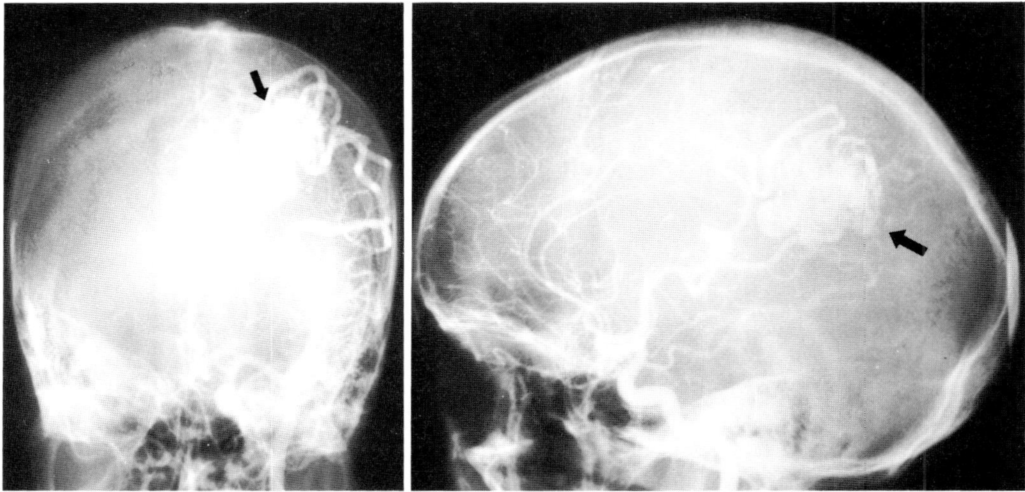

The patient was seen just after his first epileptic fit. Upon examination he was conscious and aware, but agnosia of the fingers and spastic hemiplegia were evident. A striking anomaly of blood vessels in the parietal region was discovered on angiograms of the left carotid artery. After their removal, this patient worked for at least seven years without evidence of a deficit.

Case 8: 41 year old male; superior basilar aneurysm **Fig. 41**

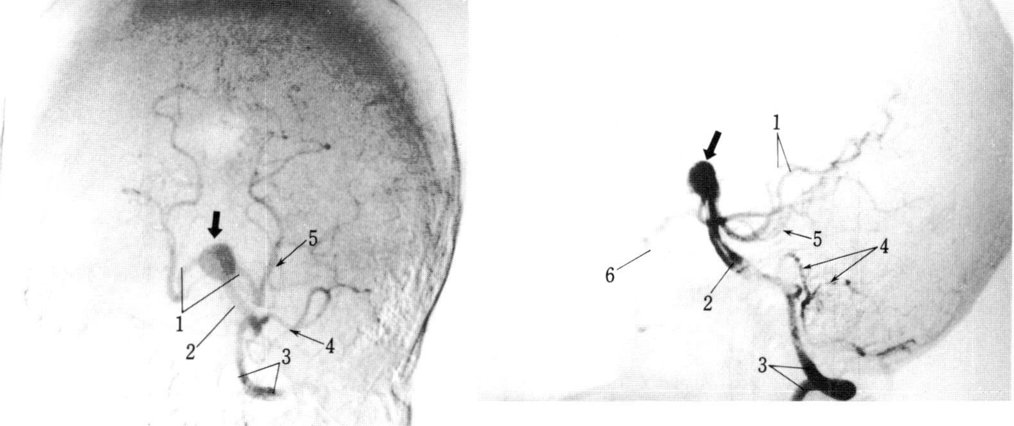

Headache was the primary complaint. CT revealed a round high absorption area in the interpeduncular cistern. No specific neurological abnormality was recognized when the patient was hospitalized, but a giant aneurysm at the top of the basilar artery was demonstrated by angiography (opacified via the basilar artery). 1) left and right posterior cerebral a.; 2) basilar a.; 3) vertebral a.; 4) posterior inferior cerebellar a.; 5) superior cerebellar a.; 6) internal carotid a.

4. THE VENTRICLES AND CEREBROSPINAL FLUID

Ventricles (Figs. 42, 43) are formed from the embryonic neural tube or spinal central canal (recall Fig. 2), which expands and transforms in the brain during development. Comparison of Fig. 43 and the last developmental stage in Fig. 2, suggests how the developing ventricular system of the embryonic brain ultimately reflects the shape of the mature cerebral hemispheres.

A lateral ventricle is located within each cerebral hemisphere (43–1 through 5). The third ventricle (43–7), Sylvian aqueduct (43–12) and fourth ventricle (43–14) are within the diencephalon, midbrain and a region formed by the pons and cerebellum, respectively. Among the various terms described in Fig. 43, three foramina, each associated with a person's name, are frequently referred to by the neurosurgeon. The first is a pair of interventricular foramina of Monro which connect the lateral ventricles with the third ventricle. The other two are foramina by which the fourth ventricle communicates with the subarachnoid space. The single foramen of Magendie (42–8) is located in the median plane and opens posteriorly. The foramen of Luschka (43–13) is paired and opens antero-laterally.

There is still some uncertainty about the specific sites of production and absorption of the cerebrospinal fluid (CSF). Most of it is definitely formed within the choroid plexus of the lateral ventricles (42–1), and flows through the third ventricle (42–5), the cerebral aqueduct (42–6), and the fourth ventricle (42–7), finally reaching the subarachnoid space by way of the foramina of Magendie and Luschka. Some CSF flows down along the spinal cord, but the majority of it circulates upward along the brain stem and subarachnoid space, thereby circling the cerebrum. The CSF finally empties into dural sinuses (42–9) by way of arachnoid villi (42–2).

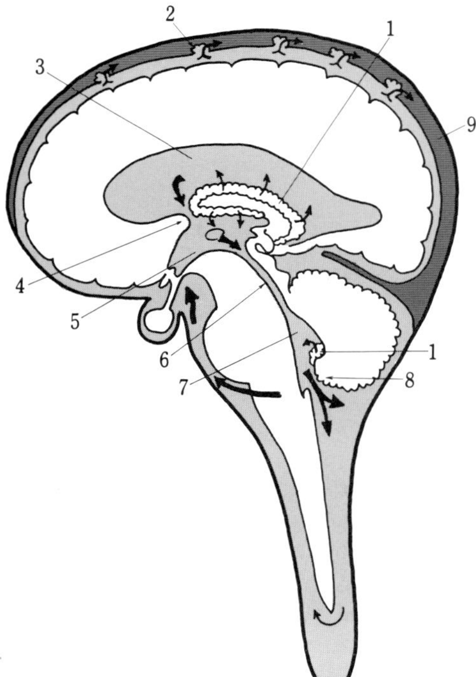

Fig. 42 Production and absorption of cerebrospinal fluid.

1. choroid plexus
2. arachnoid granulation
3. lateral ventricle
4. foramen of Monro
5. third ventricle
6. cerebral aqueduct
7. fourth ventricle
8. foramen of Magendie
9. superior sagittal sinus

Ventricular drainage and shunting operations usually involve the puncturing of a lateral ventricle. A lumbar puncture into the lumbar subarachnoid space provides information about cerebrospinal fluid pressure and certain pathologic conditions (inflammation, subarachnoid hemorrhage), because the CSF within the subarachnoid space around the spinal cord normally communicates with the CSF in the cranium. The CSF has a protective role because of its buoyant effect and waste-removal function. When the circulation of this fluid is impeded, it remains trapped within the ventricles, such that its pressure rises and ultimately creates a condition known as hydrocephalus.

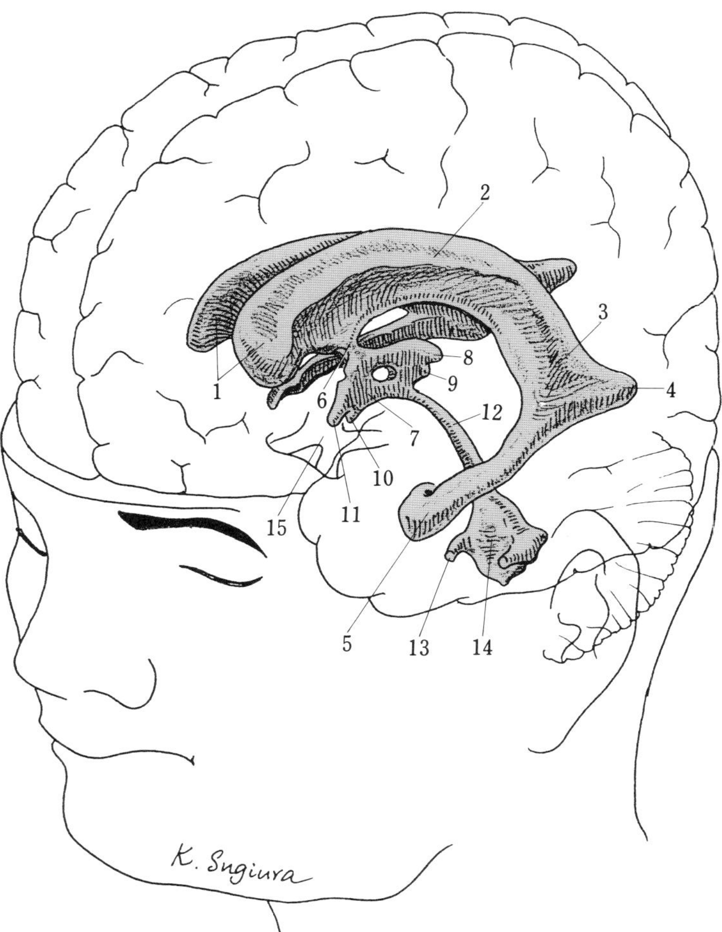

Fig. 43 A three-dimensional representation of the ventricular system.

1. anterior horn of the lateral ventricle
2. body of the lateral ventricle
3. collateral trigone of the lateral ventricle
4. posterior horn of the lateral ventricle
5. temporal horn of the lateral ventricle
6. foramen of Monro
7. third ventricle
8. suprapineal recess
9. pineal recess
10. infundibular recess
11. optic recess
12. cerebral aqueduct (of Sylvius)
13. foramen of Luschka
14. fourth ventricle
15. chiasma

INTRACRANIAL PNEUMOGRAPHY

An X-ray technique, now obsolete, used air or oxygen as a contrast medium for visualizing the brain and surrounding structures, such as the ventricles and the subarachnoid space.

In 1912, Luckette found, while looking at an X-ray, that air had entered the ventricles of a traumatized patient. This observation occured at about the same time as the first clinician, W.E. Dandy, attempted to inject air into the human brain for diagnostic purposes. He developed both pneumoventriculography (PVG; 1918), in which air was directly injected into the ventricles and, subsequently, pneumoencephalography (PEG), in which air was injected into the lumbar subarachnoid space.

Dandy preferred PEG, but, like all subsequent researchers and clinicians, used PVG when increased intracranial pressure was evident. The introduction of the fractional technique in 1940, made PEG much less dangerous, when done carefully. However, danger and pain could not be fully obviated. With the introduction of CT and, more recently, magnetic resonance imaging, PEG is no longer performed. In PVG and PEG no single film reveals the ventricles in their entirety. Rather, their full visualization requires a number of X-ray films, taken successively as the air travels upwards into locations selected by changing the position of the head (Figs. 44–45).

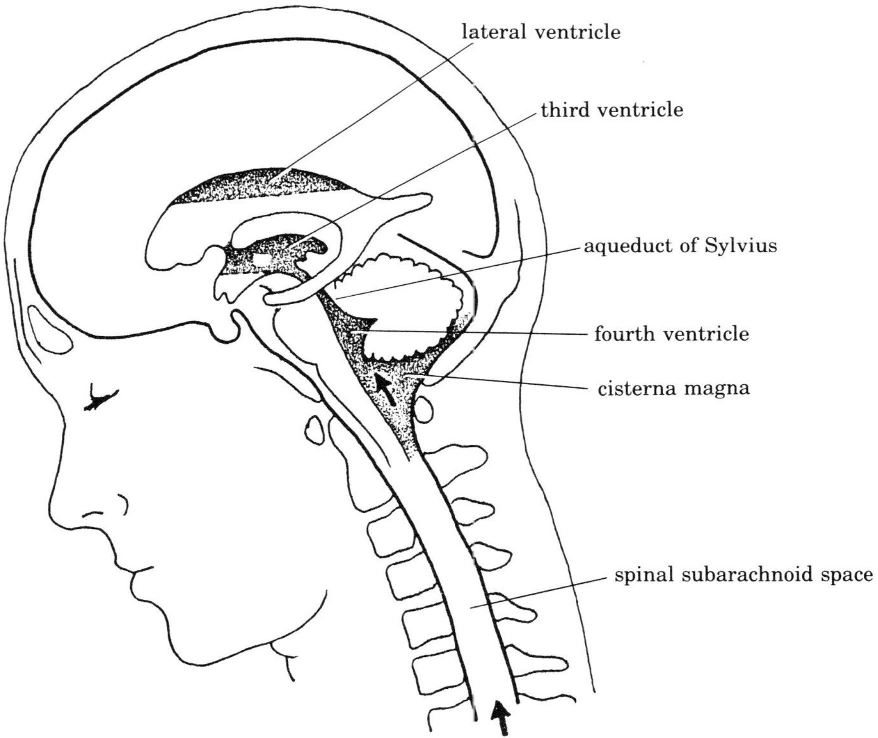

Fig. 44 Pathways and air pooling in pneumoencephalography.
With the patient sitting in a forward-bending posture, injected air travels from the spinal cord subarachnoid space to the cisterna magna, through the foramen of Magendie into the fourth ventricle, through the cerebral aqueduct to the third ventricle, through the foramina of Monro, and finally into the lateral ventricles.

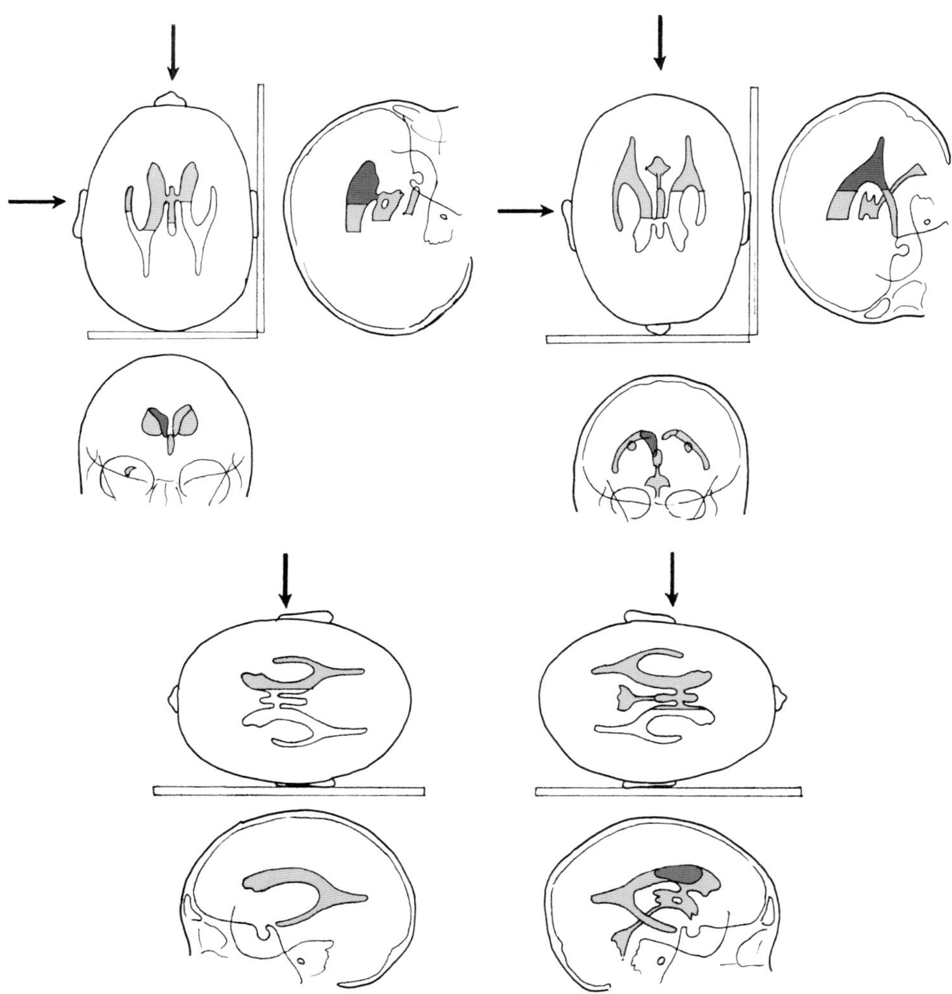

Fig. 45 Normal ventricular shapes revealed by different positions of the head.

All the parts of the ventricular system cannot appear in a single film. Rather, several films must be viewed to form an image of the ventricles in their entirety.

In addition to the ventricles, cisterns and the subarachnoid space are revealed by PEG. Cisterns are expansions of the subarachnoid space (Fig. 46). Their identification is essential when reading a pneumoencephalogram.

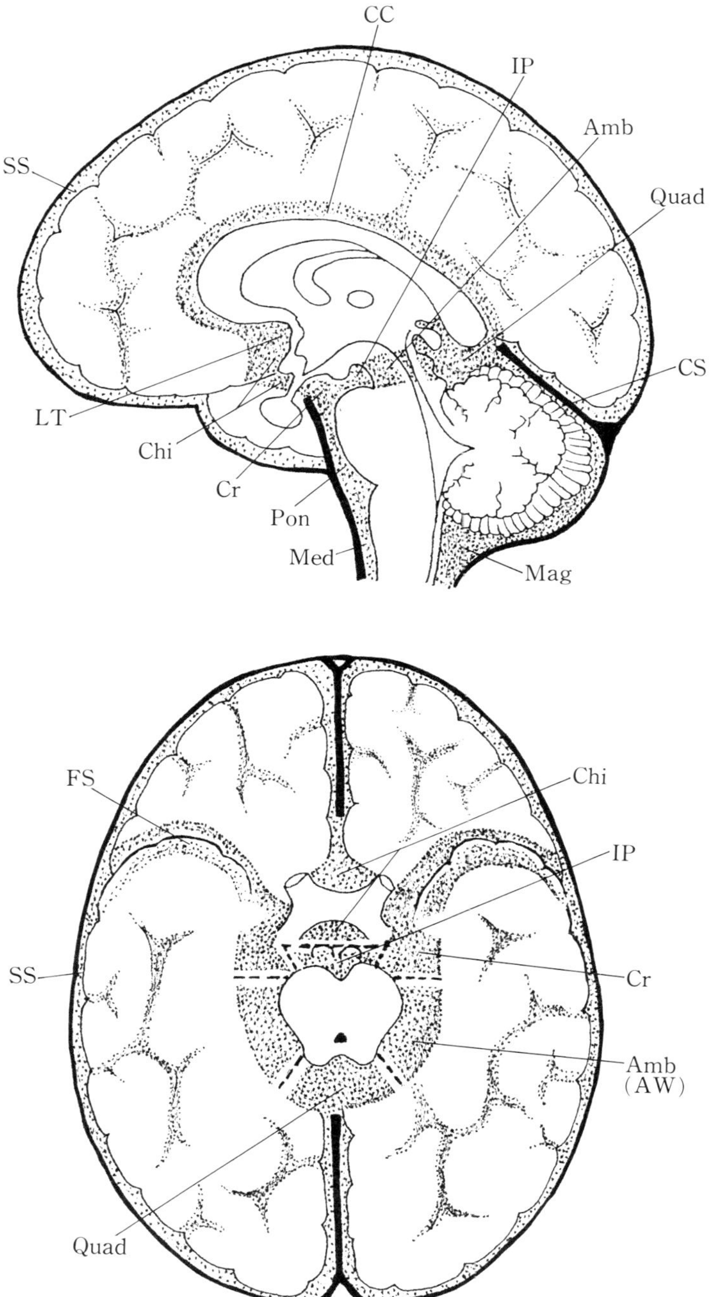

Fig. 46 Nomenclature and locations of cisterns.

Amb: ambient cistern
AW: ambient wing cistern
CC: cisterna corporis callosi
Chi: chiasmatic cistern
Cr: crural cistern
CS: cisterna cerebelli superior
FS: cisterna fissurae Sylvii
IP: interpeduncular cistern
LT: cisterna laminae terminalis
Mag: cisterna magna
Med: medullary cistern
Pon: pontine cistern
Quad: quadrigeminal cistern
SS: subarachnoid space

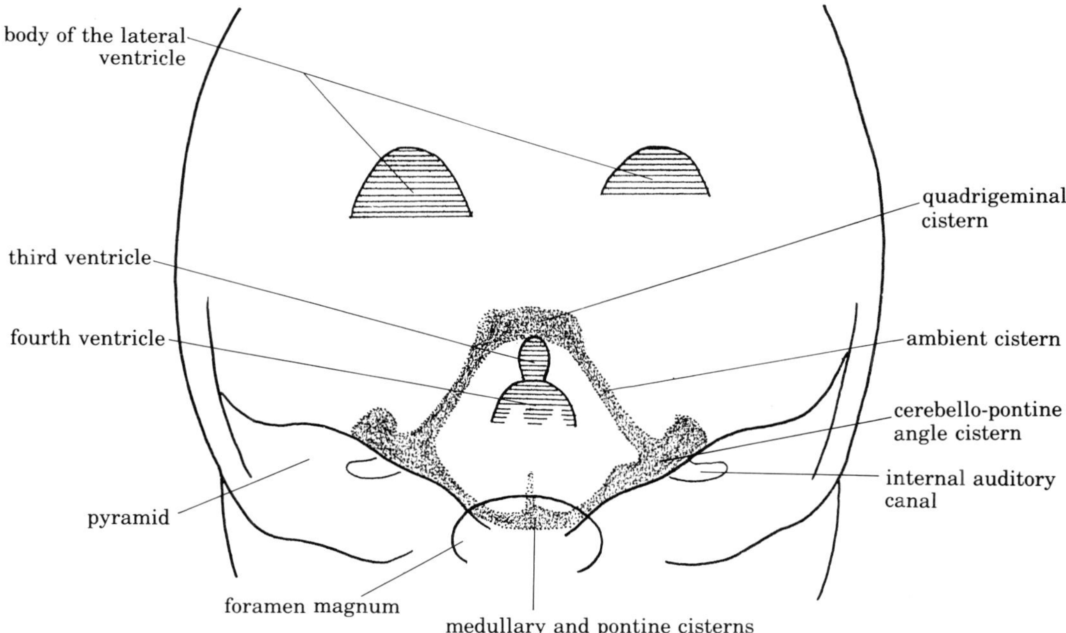

Fig. 47 A diagram derived from a normal pneumoencephalogram, taken during air injection in the sitting position; antero-posterior view.

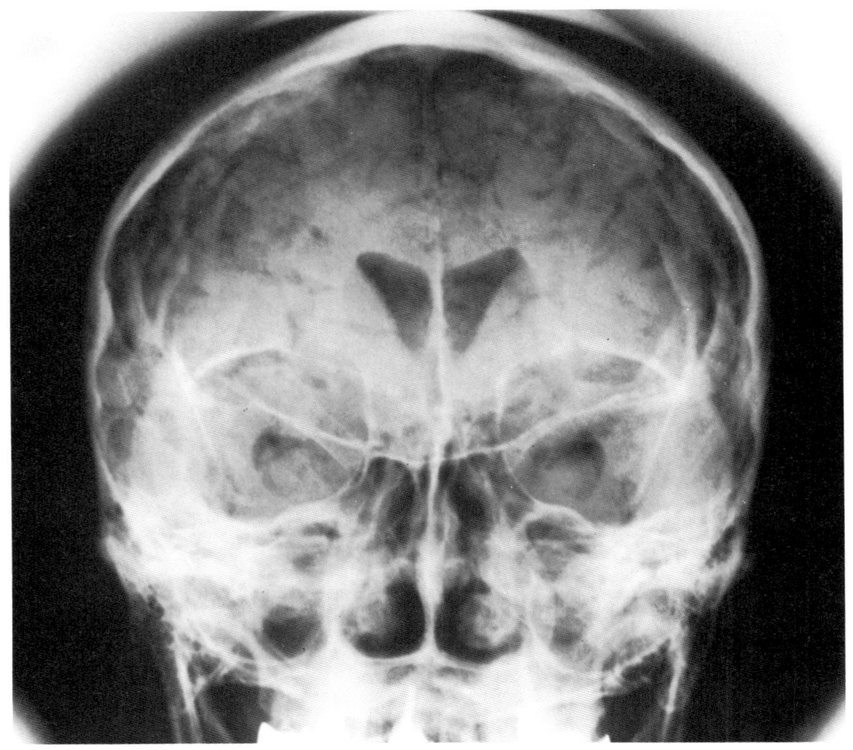

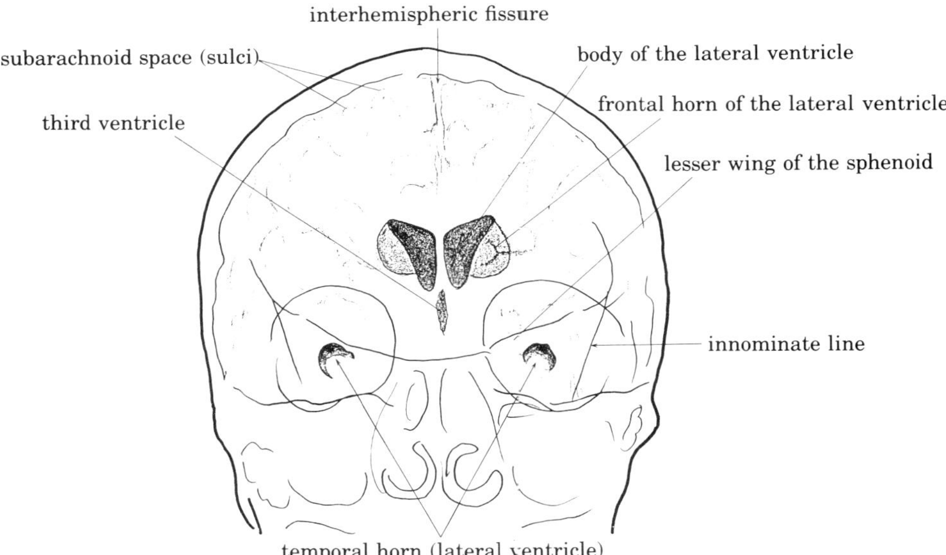

Fig. 48 A normal pneumoencephalogram taken in the supine, brow-up position; antero-posterior view.

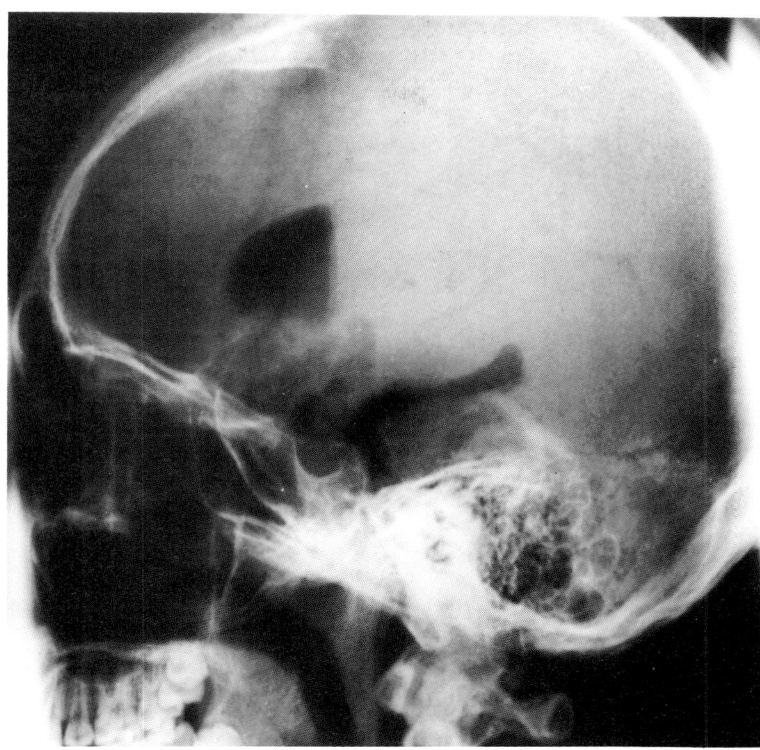

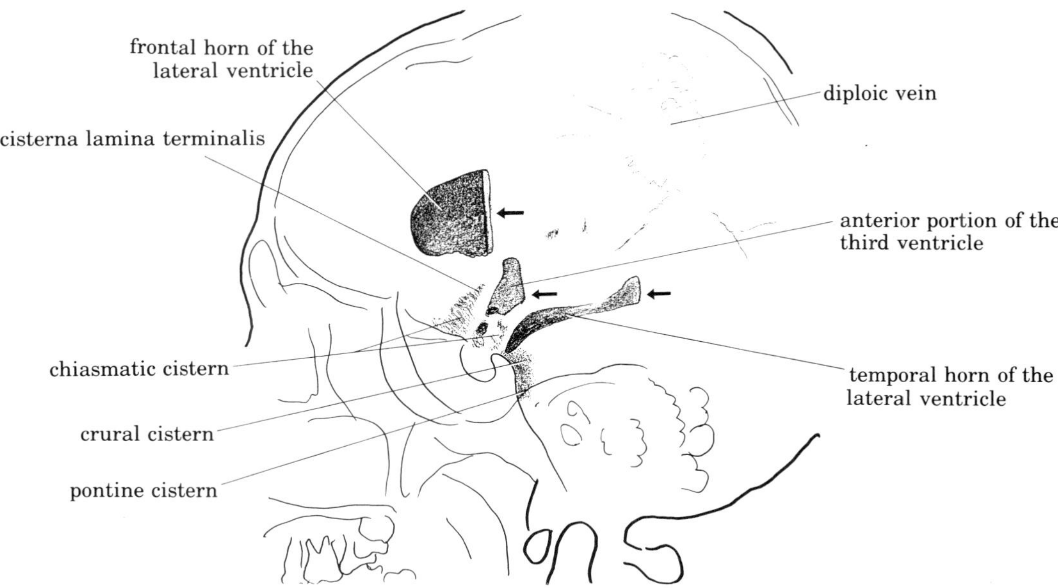

Fig. 49 A normal pneumoencephalogram taken in the supine, brow-up position; lateral view.
Note the niveau (←) revealed in a lateral view.

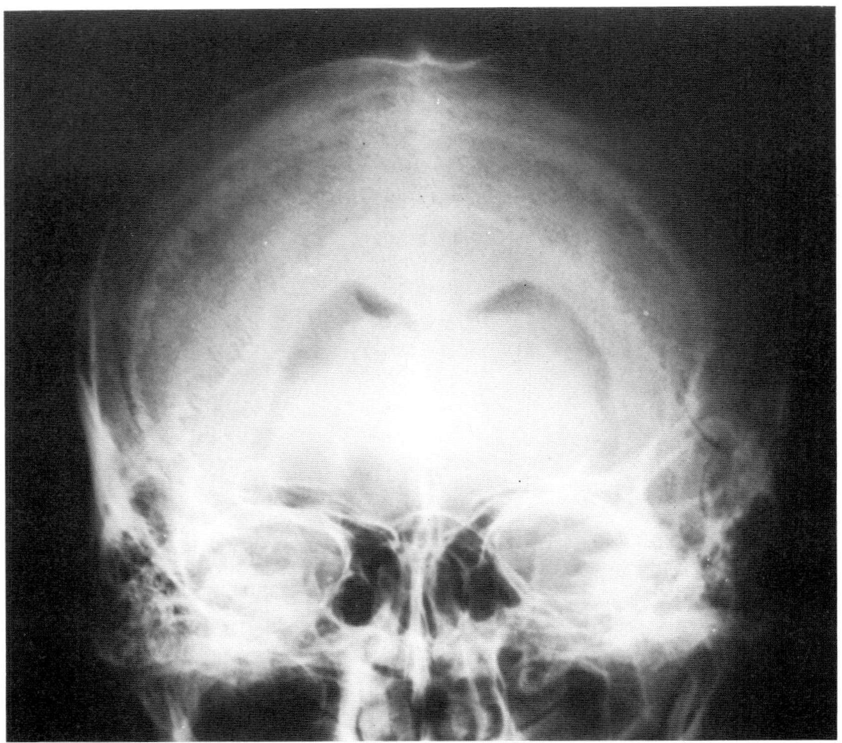

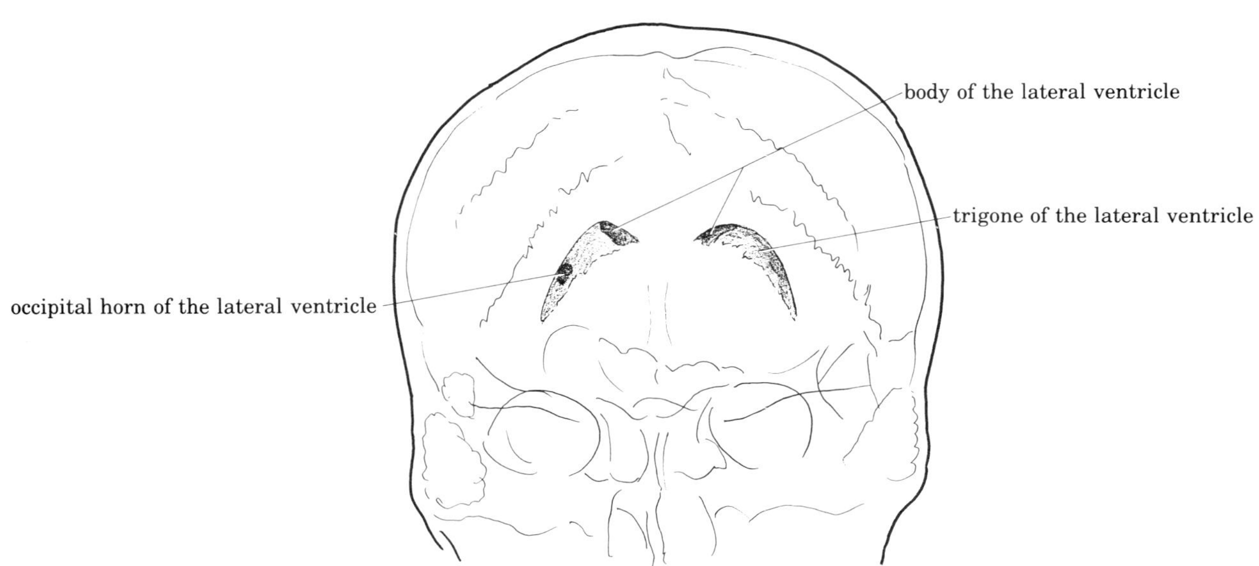

Fig. 50 A normal pneumoencephalogram taken in the prone, brow-down position; postero-anterior view.

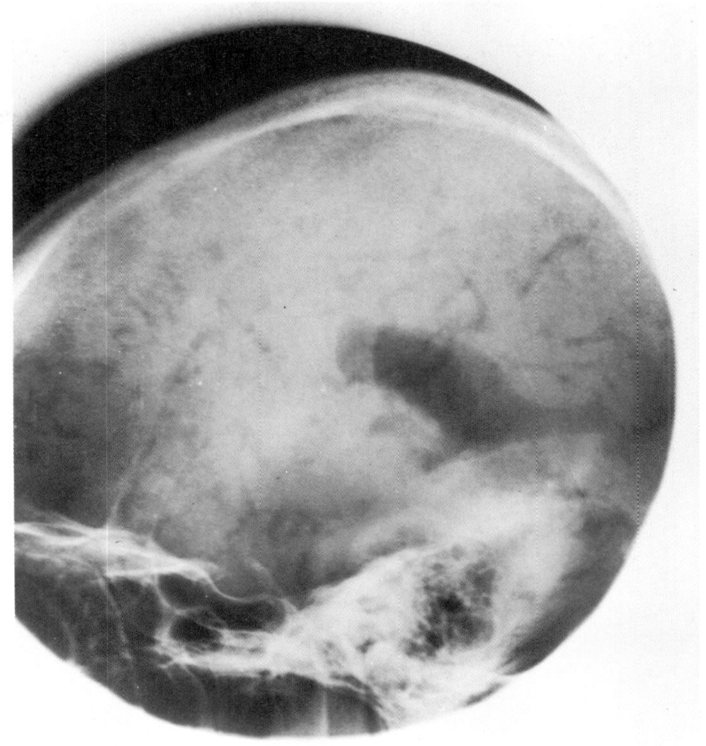

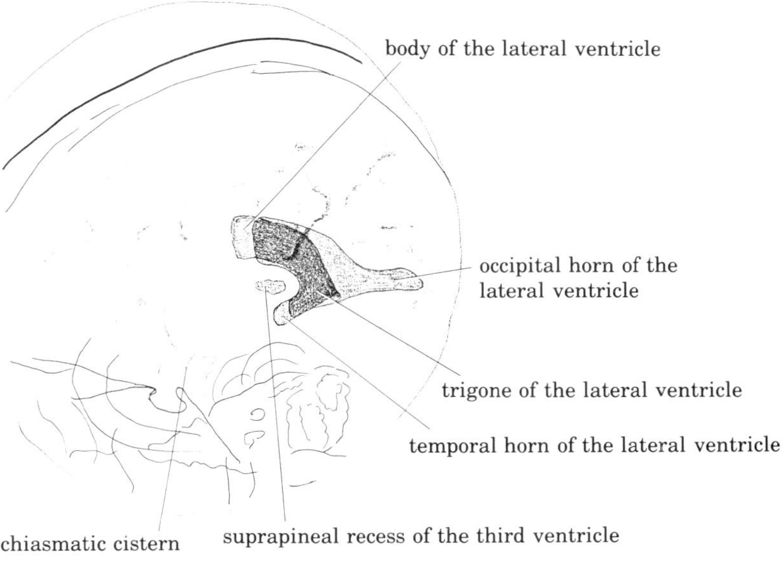

Fig. 51 A normal pneumoencephalogram taken in the prone, brow-down position; lateral view.

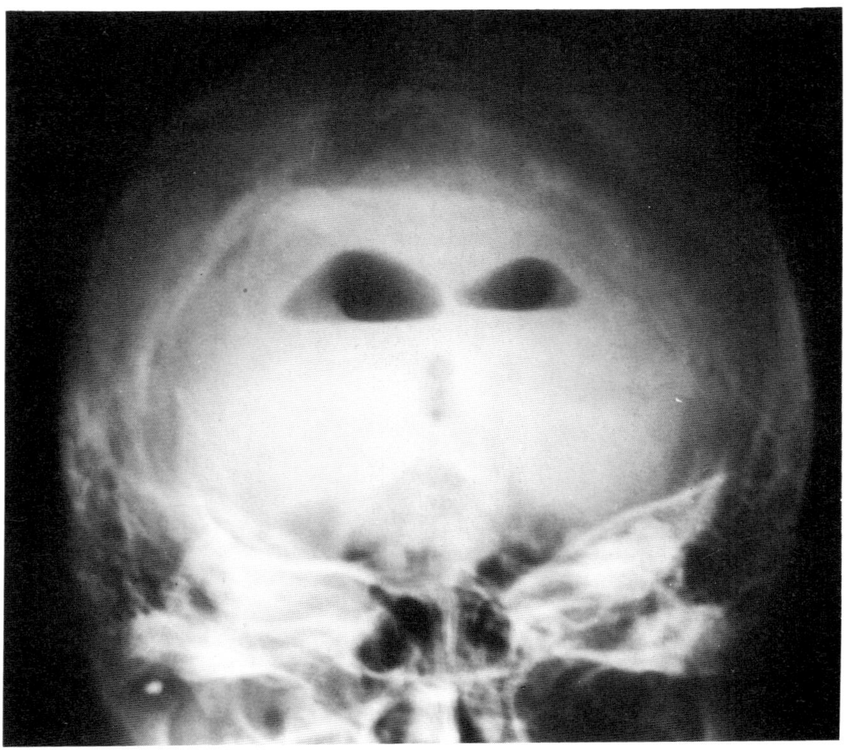

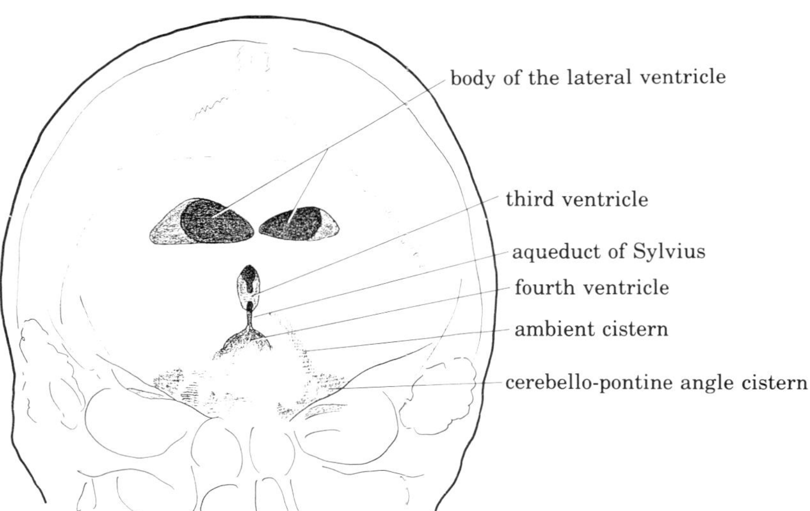

Fig. 52 A normal pneumoencephalogram taken in the sitting position with the head bending forward; postero-anterior view.

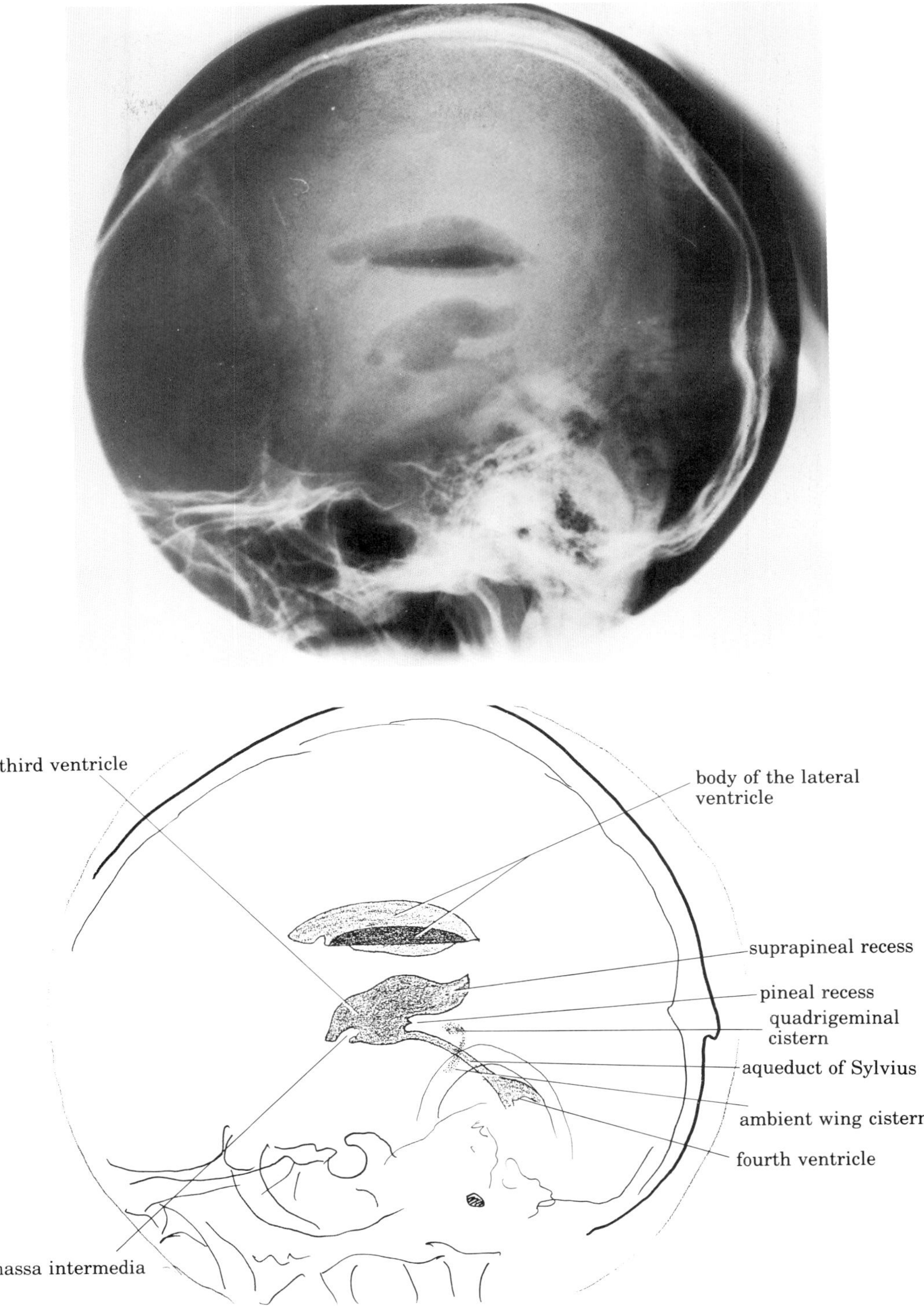

Fig. 53 A normal pneumoencephalogram taken in the sitting position, with the head bending forward; lateral view.

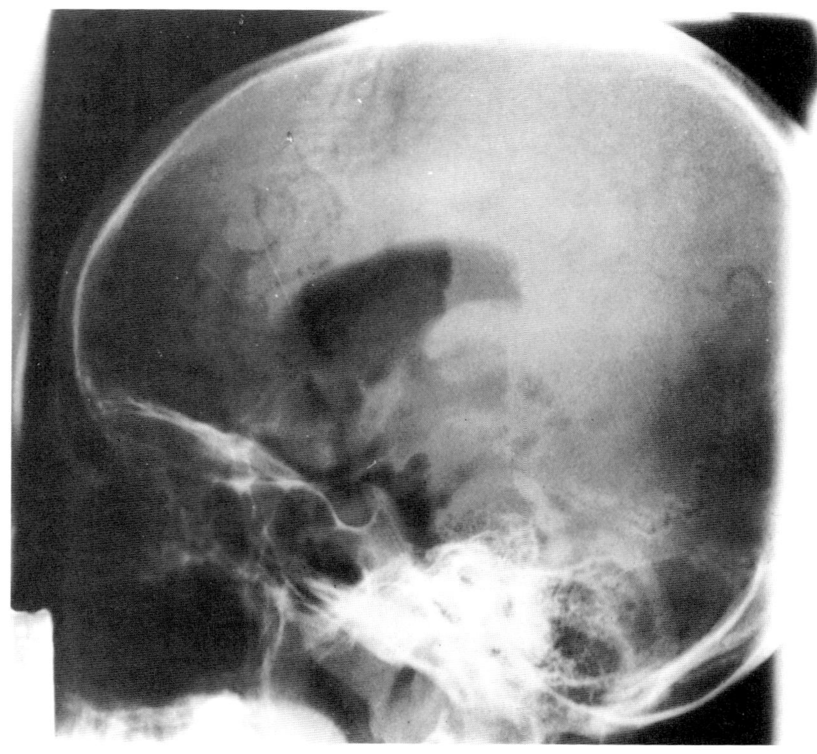

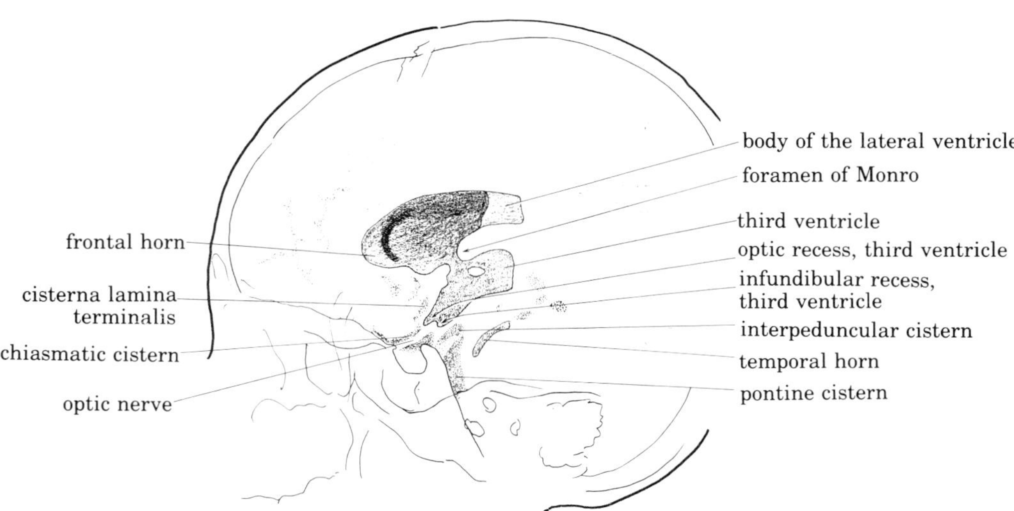

Fig. 54 A normal pneumoencephalogram taken in the supine, brow-up position; lateral view.

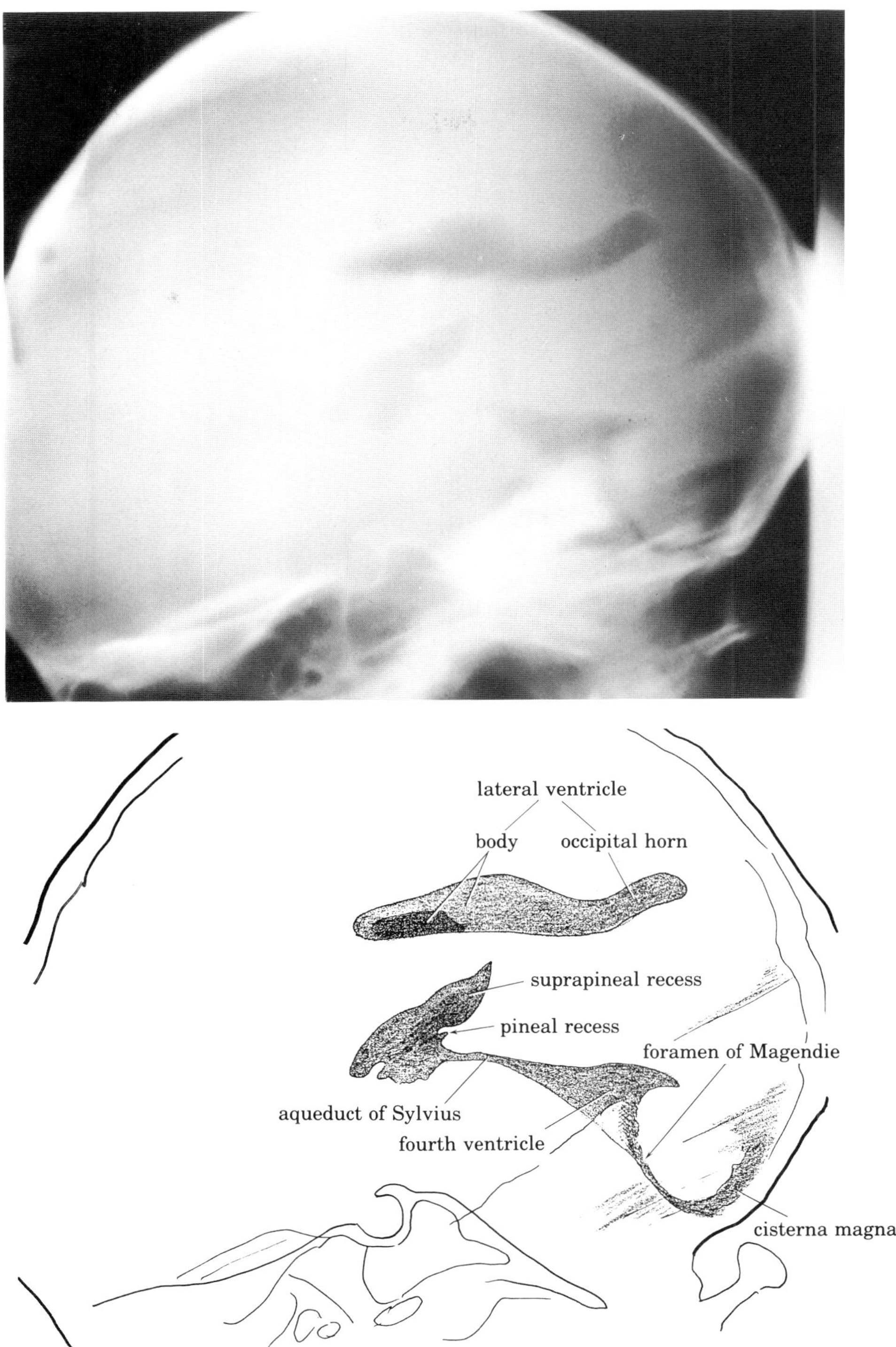

Fig. 55 Use of tomography in the sitting position; normal lateral view. With the use of tomography, structures in the mid-sagittal plane become clearer than in a conventional pneumoencephalogram (cf. Fig. 53).

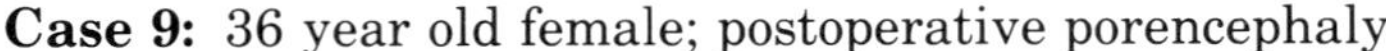

Case 9: 36 year old female; postoperative porencephaly

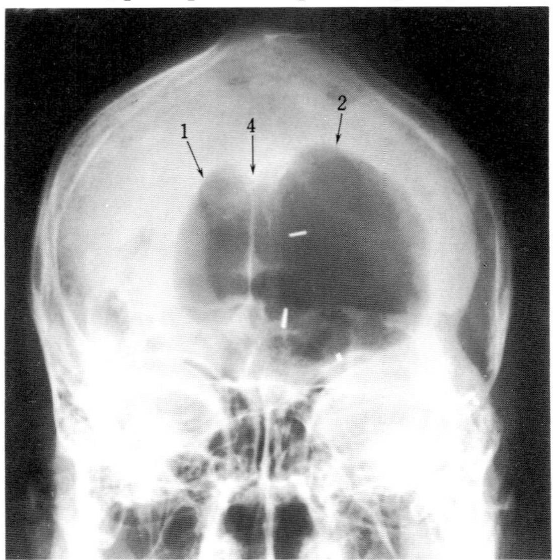

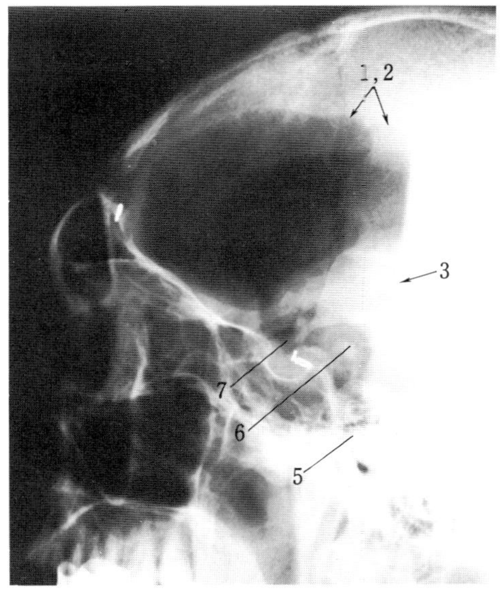

Fig. 56

An anomaly of blood vessels in the left frontal lobe had been removed a year before the examination. The left and right lateral ventricles and the third ventricle had expanded. In particular, the left lateral ventricle was enlarged and it communicated with a space formed in the frontal lobe. 1) right lateral ventricle; 2) left lateral ventricle; 3) third ventricle; 4) septum pellucidum; 5) pontine cistern; 6) interpeduncular cistern; 7) cistern of the chiasma.

Case 10: 25 year old female; ependymoma within the fourth ventricle

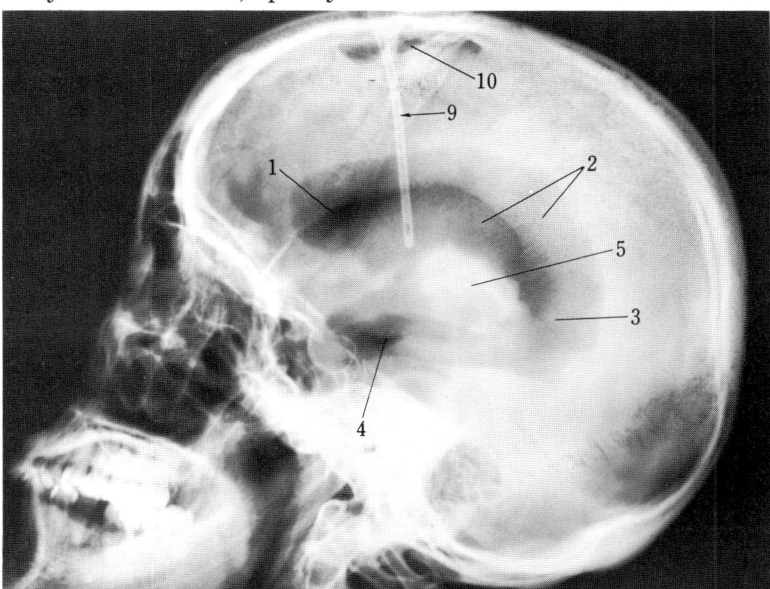

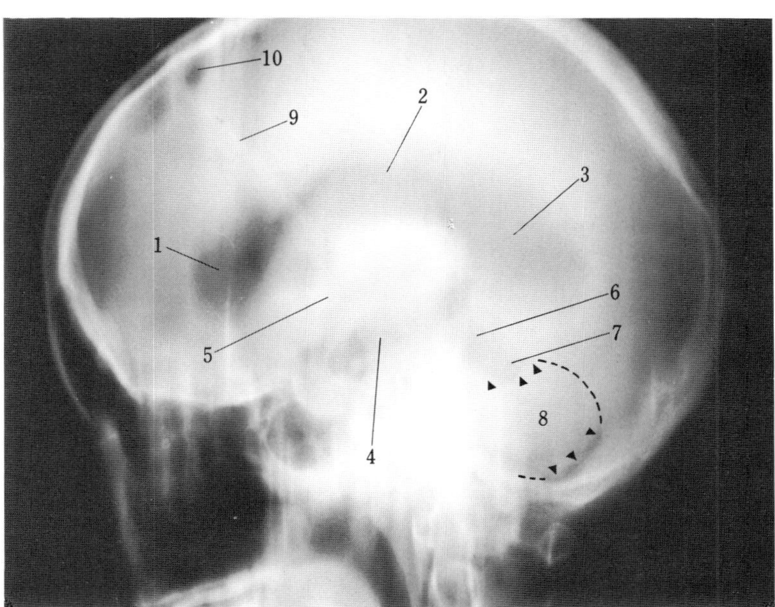

Fig. 57

Primary complaints were headache, vomiting and impaired walking. Papilledema and ataxia of the extremities were also evident. Pneumography was done by inserting a tube (9) through a hole (10) drilled in the frontal bone. The lateral ventricles (1–4), third ventricle (5) and cerebral aqueduct (6) appeared to be expanded. Note that the tumor (8) which was seen at surgery had swollen to displace the fourth ventricle (7).

5. TOPOGRAPHICAL ANATOMY OF THE BRAIN AND SELECTED LOCAL FEATURES

BRAIN TOPOGRAPHY

The surface of the brain is generally divided into four lobes, termed frontal (58–1), temporal (58–2), parietal (58–3) and occipital (58–4). Each lobe's surface is folded and convoluted. Each ridge is called a gyrus (pl., gyri), and each groove between them is called a sulcus (pl., sulci). Sulci display considerable individual variability, but three of them are normally recognizable across subjects: 1) the lateral sulcus (fissure of Sylvius) (58–5), 2) the central sulcus (sulcus of Rolando) (58–6) and 3) the calcarine sulcus (58–7).

The boundaries between the cerebral lobes are not always clear cut, except for those between the frontal and parietal lobes (divided by the central sulcus) and between the temporal and frontal or parietal lobes (divided by the fissure of Sylvius).

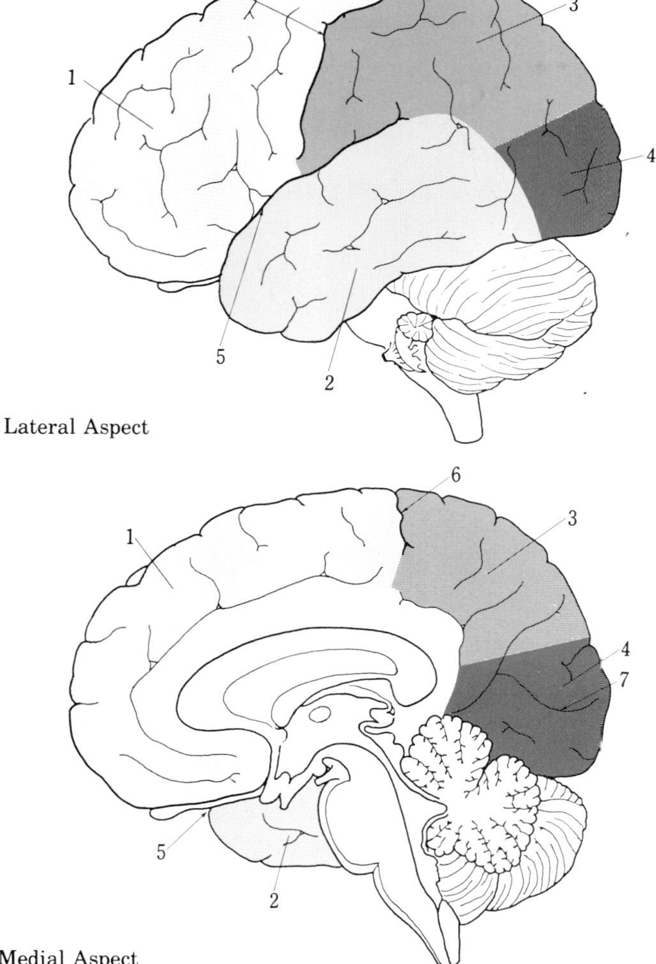

Fig. 58 The sulci and lobes of the brain.

1. frontal lobe
2. temporal lobe
3. parietal lobe
4. occipital lobe
5. lateral sulcus (fissure of Sylvius)
6. central sulcus (of Rolando)
7. calcarine sulcus

There is another lobe called the insula (of Reil) which cannot be seen on the brain's surface. This triangle-shaped structure (Figs. 59, 60) is covered by the operculum (60–2) deep within the fissure of Sylvius. The functions of the insula are not described here. However, its recognition is essential when reading angiograms. It is also an important guide during a procedure where direct removal of an intracerebral hematoma is attempted.

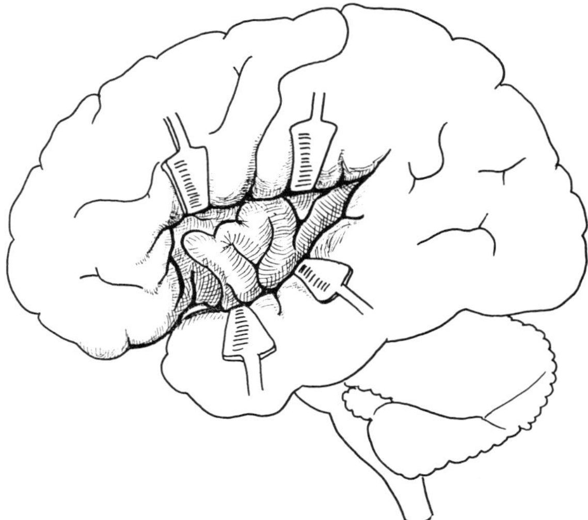

Fig. 59 Diagram showing how the insula is revealed by opening the fissure of Sylvius.

Thick branches of the middle cerebral artery (Sylvian group) run on the surface of the insula and help delineate its triangular shape.

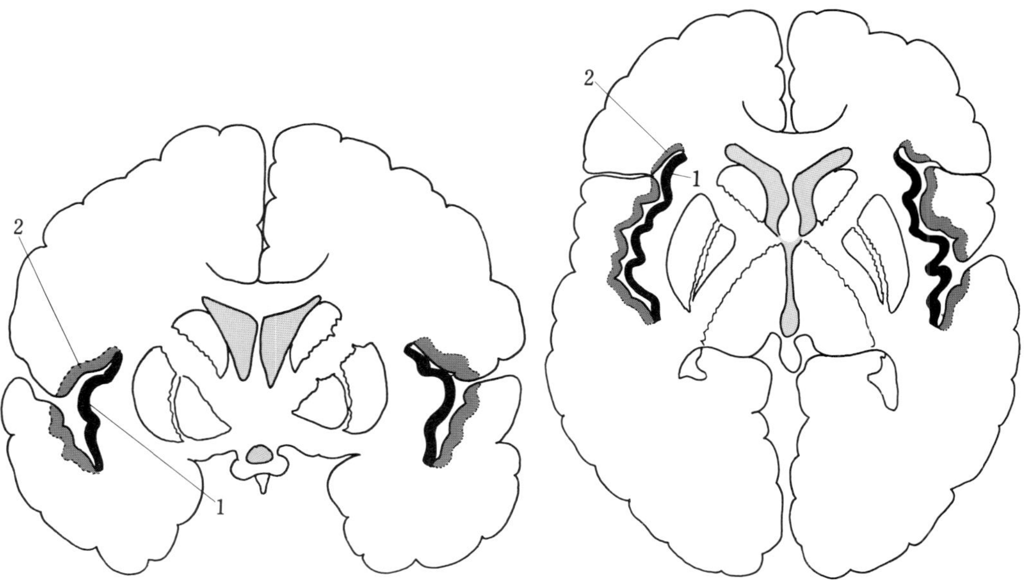

Fig. 60 The insula and operculum.

1. insula (Reil) 2. operculum

FRONTAL LOBE

At a first approximation, the frontal lobe subserves; 1) motor functions (voluntary and involuntary), 2) mental functions (emotion, insight, personality, etc.) and 3) motor aspects of speech production. The motor area is located in front of the central sulcus (of Rolando). Immediately anterior to this sulcus lies area 4 of Brodmann (Fig. 61) which is implicated in command signals for movement. The cortical areas with connections to specific body parts are shown in Fig. 62–A. The body parts that generally engage in relatively coarse movements (thorax, abdomen, proximal parts of extremities) do not require a large projection from their corresponding cortical areas. On the other hand, the body parts which engage in finely controlled movements have a relatively larger cortical representation. Motor fibers from this area contribute to the pyramidal tract which projects to brain stem and spinal motor nuclei as well as adjacent parts of the anterior horn of the spinal cord. A lesion in or close to the motor area causes a focal paralysis of the face, hands or feet (monoplegia), depending on the specific site of damage. If the motor area is stimulated, a particular type of fit, called Jacksonian epilepsy is generated. It begins in a restricted body part and gradually spreads to the entire body.

Areas 6 and 8 (Fig. 61) in front of area 4, are also important for the control of movement. Damage to these areas causes abnormal involuntary movements and increased muscle tonus, which impairs the smooth execution of voluntary movements.

Area 8 is called the area of eye movements because it plays an important role in regulating the cooperative movement of both eye balls. When area 8 on the left side is abnormally stimulated (as in epilepsy) the eye balls turn to the right (healthy side). On the other hand, when this area is damaged by hemorrhage, the function of the contralateral area 8 becomes predominant and the eye balls turn to the left (damaged side). This phenomenon is called conjugate deviation.

Located antero-inferiorly to area 4 is the motor speech center (Brodmann's area 44) in the left hemisphere. This region is called Broca's speech center. Since the inferior end of area 4 helps control tongue, mouth and throat movements, it seems appropriate that the motor speech area should lie immediately ahead of this area. A lesion of the motor speech area causes motor dysphasia. The patient understands what is spoken, but loses smooth control of the tongue, mouth and throat. Consequently they cannot speak. The sensory speech center (of Wernicke) is also located in the left temporal lobe. It must never be compromised during an operation on the left side of the brain.

Frontal lobe tissues other than those mentioned above are often called silent areas because direct damage is not followed by obvious symptoms, such as paralysis or dysphasia. However, this does not mean that these silent areas have no function. On the inferior surface of the frontal lobe lies an area controlling higher mental functions, easily demonstrated in human beings. As a lesion begins in this area, the patient loses intellectual capacity and personality. As the lesion enlarges, the patient loses the capacity for emotional display, their social and moral values deteriorate and, finally, they pay little attention to previous interests and lose the ability to react appropriately to various circumstances. These deficits are also displayed after a frontal lobotomy, a once-popular operation for patients with various mental dysfunctions, including hyper-anxious states.

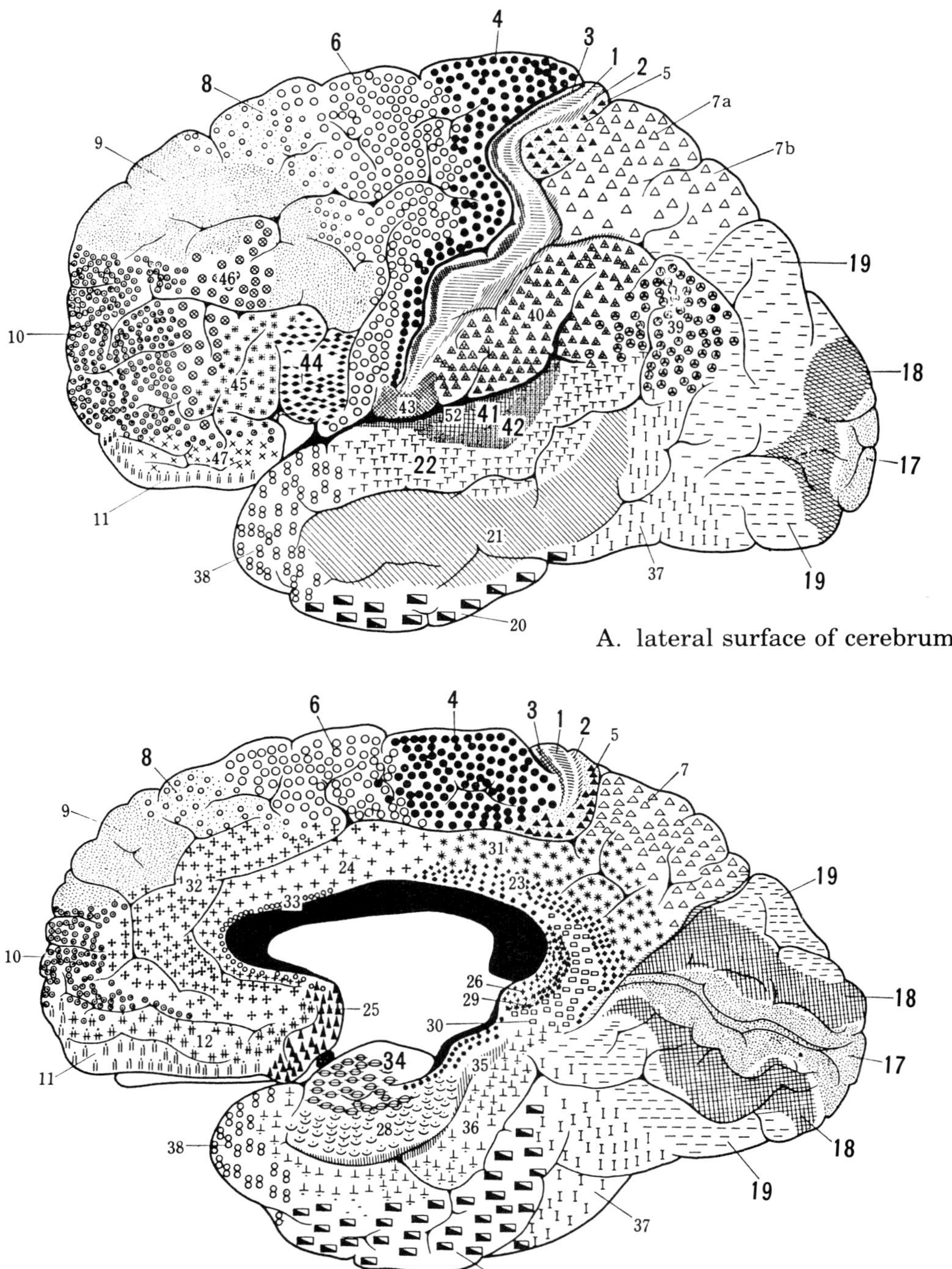

Fig. 61 Brodmann's anatomically defined areas of the human cerebral cortex.

It is time consuming to memorize each number in Brodmann's scheme. However, they are frequently cited in neurology textbooks. Certainly, the boldfaced numbers in this figure (showing particularly important areas) should be memorized.

PARIETAL LOBE

This lobe has numerous centers. The senses of heat, cold, touch, pain and so forth are called somatic senses. These are represented by sensory receptive areas behind the central sulcus (Fig. 61; areas 1, 2, 3). Sensory information from various parts of the body is conducted to particular locations within these areas (Fig. 62–B), in a fashion similar to that for the motor area (Fig. 62–A).

The remainder of the parietal cortex contributes to complex functions. For example, a disturbance of the nondominant hemisphere (usually the right side) causes spatial agnosia, involving loss of orientation by the individual in space and in time. A patient with a cerebral tumor in the right parietal lobe might lose their way when travelling to the office in which they have worked for many years. Similarly, they might get lost in their own house, when looking for a particular room.

A well-known disorder of the dominant hemisphere (left) is Gerstmann syndrome. This is a combination of finger agnosia, right-left disorientation, agraphia, acalculia and so on. In the case of finger agnosia, the patient cannot distinguish their fingers, particularly when they are concealed from them. When asked to lift up the forefinger, the patient might lift the little finger or twist the head to see the fingers. In right-left disorientation, the patient loses the ability to distinguish between the right and left sides of his body. If asked to touch the right ear with the left hand, they

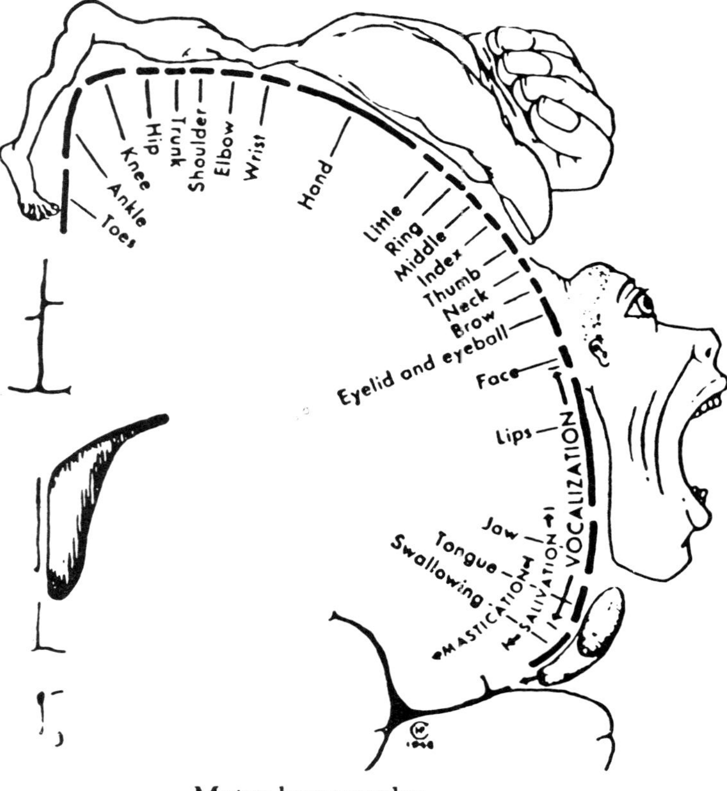

Fig. 62 Cortical distribution of functions according to Penfield and Rasmussen.
A. Cortical location of motor functions

might do nothing or, alternately, they might make an incorrect right-left distinction. Agraphia is the loss of writing ability, and acalculia is the inability to make even the simplest of arithmetic calculations. These symptoms are all due to disorders of complicated senses.

Other symptoms of parietal-lobe disturbances include apraxia, astereognosia and loss of body image. In apraxia, movements are not executed in the right order. For example, when given matches and cigarettes, the patient might hold a match in the mouth and try to light it with a cigarette. Astereognosia is the loss of ability to discriminate the shape of an object on the basis of sensory input from the fingers, and loss of the memory of the relationship between a particular input and a particular object. Loss of body image involves nonrecognition of the side of the body contralateral to the damaged parietal lobe (usually on the non-dominant side). The patient feels that half of the body has disappeared, or that it belongs to someone else.

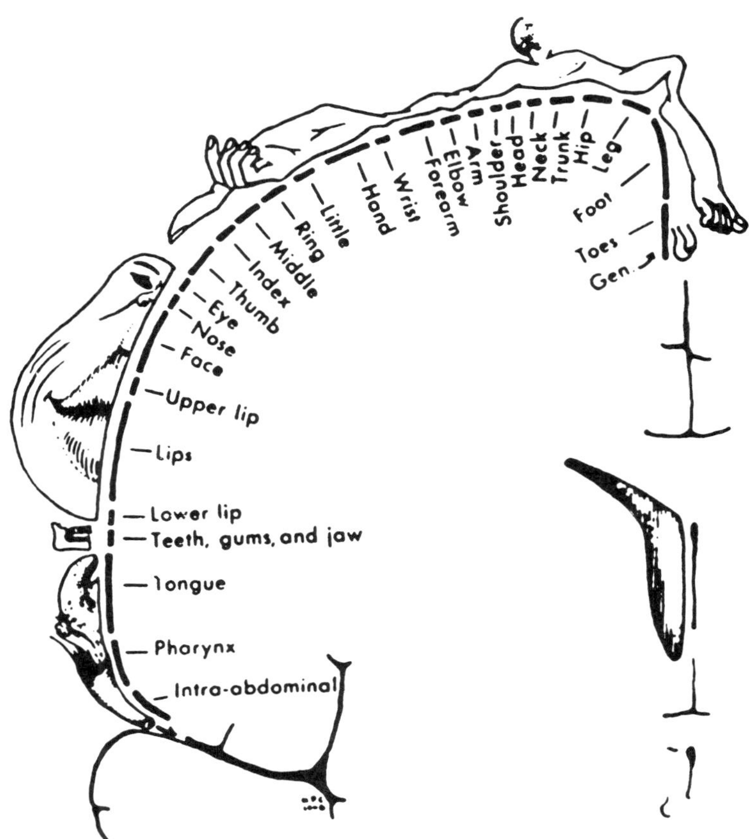

Sensory homunculus

Fig. 62B Cortical location of sensory functions.

Although Fig. 62 is separated into two parts, the motor (A) and sensory (B) representations are quite similar. Frequent review of these figures will aid in the understanding of clinical signs. For example, paraparesis of the legs results from a lesion located supero-medially in both hemispheres (occurring, e.g., with a parasagittal meningioma).

TEMPORAL LOBE

The temporal lobe includes centers for hearing, smell, memory and speech. It also forms a part of the limbic system.

The center for hearing is located in Heschl's gyrus (Fig. 61; areas 41–42) close to the fissure of Sylvius. Stimulation of this cortical area generates an acoustic spasm (acouasm). In cases of its damage, cortical deafness and hearing agnosia may occur.

The sensory speech center of Wernicke in the left (dominant) hemisphere is just posterior to the center for hearing (Fig. 61; posterior to area 22). A lesion in this region causes sensory dysphasia. In a pure case, the patient cannot understand what is spoken to them, even though their hearing is normal; just as if they are hearing a foreign language for the first time. This is the reason why neurosurgeons stay well away from the left superior temporal gyrus, especially its posterior portion.

The center for smell is said to be within the uncus on the medial under surface of the temporal lobe (Fig. 61; area 34). A dreamy state can result from temporal lobe epilepsy. The patient may experience an inexplicably unpleasant smell. This is the well-known uncinate fit, as pointed out by Jackson.

The center for memory is thought to be in or around the hippocampus, located inferior and medial to the temporal lobe. If this region is disturbed, the patient has difficulty in recalling events they should indeed remember. Patients also experience a sensory abnormality called deja vu (Fr., 'already seen') involving the feeling that an object presented for the first time has been previously seen.

The hippocampus and uncus also have important functions as part of the limbic system (described later). For example, a bilateral disturbance of the temporal lobe can cause Kluver-Bucy syndrome* in addition to the deficits described above.

OCCIPITAL LOBE

The center for vision is located on the medial surface of the occipital lobe surrounding the calcarine sulcus (Fig. 61; area 17). Information concerning an object in the right side of the visual field passes through the optic nerve, optic chiasma, optic tract, lateral geniculate body and optic radiation, to finally reach the left visual receptive area where the process of visual perception begins. A lesion of the occipital lobe causes homonymous hemianopia of the contralateral side (a lesion of the left side causes a hemianopia on the right side). The central portion of the visual field is not disturbed in this particular case (macular sparing).

There are association areas above and below the center for vision (Fig. 61; areas 18–19) relating to visual perception. Following lesions in these areas, objects are seen, but their significance is not appreciated. For example, a patient might see a ballpoint pen, but not realize that it is a tool for writing (visual agnosia).

A center for the control of eye movements is located in area 19. It modulates visual reflexes mediated largely by the superior colliculus.

---

*A syndrome seen in a monkey following bilateral destruction of the temporal lobes. Typical clinical cases are rare. The symptoms include visual agnosia, the tendency to place all presented objects in the mouth and disturbances of emotion, sexual behavior and food preference.

LIMBIC SYSTEM

The concept of a limbic system is based on a group of seemingly related functions. As a result, textbooks differ in their interpretation of the specific components of this system. However, they all agree that these components are scattered widely throughout the brain (Fig. 63) and that they function by virtue of their connections with one another.

For functional reasons, the limbic system is also called the visceral brain or emotional brain. Its main functions involve emotional expression like pleasure, excitement, anger, fear and discomfort. It also contributes to the control of visceral activity by way of the hypothalamus.

Some specific anecdotes about limbic function are now presented. It is usually very enjoyable to see a comedy. Information from the eyes and ears is directed to their respective sensory centers through intermediate nuclei in the thalamus. In-parallel and subsequent projections also project to the frontal lobe and limbic system. The end result is the experience that the comedy is funny. Alternatively, suppose a patient suffers heavily from gallstone colic. Noxious input from the gallbladder is conducted to the parietal lobe and also to the limbic system, some by way of the frontal lobe. This sensory input and central processing forces the patient to realize that the body is in a very uncomfortable state. What happens if the comedy is seen again? Even if it is equally funny, the limbic system would deprive all sensation of fun.

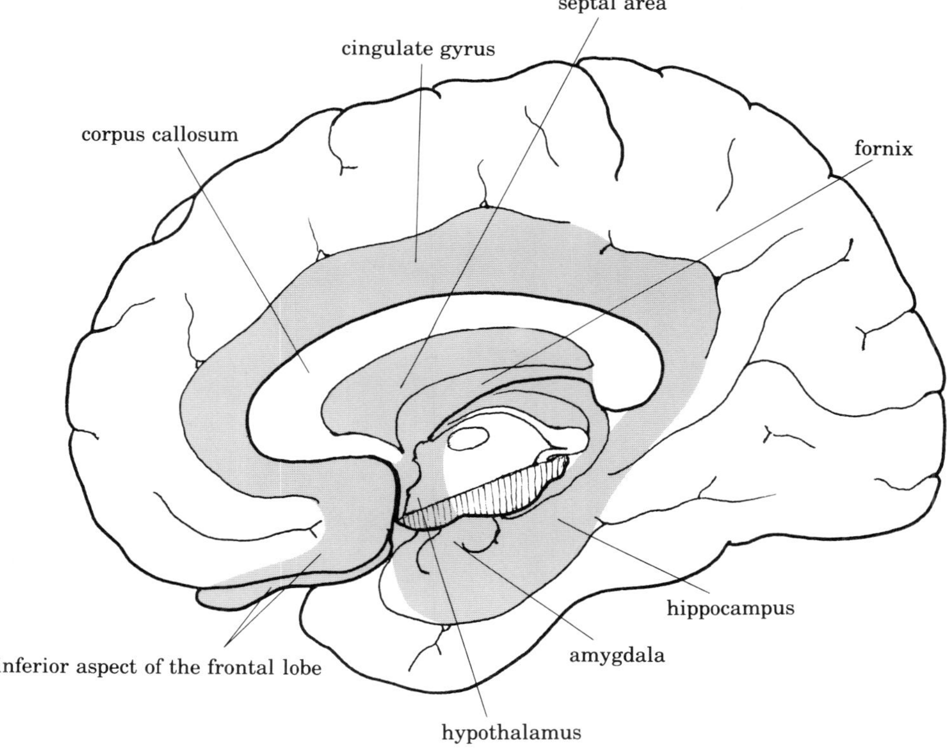

Fig. 63 Components of the limbic system.

BASAL GANGLIA

The basal ganglia is a general term incorporating the caudate nucleus, putamen, globus pallidus and subthalamic nuclei (body of Luys). The red nucleus and substantia nigra in the midbrain are sometimes added to the list. Together the caudate nucleus and putamen are called the corpus striatum, while the putamen and globus pallidus form the nucleus lenticularis. Before memorizing these names, it is helpful to recognize their location, shape and function.

The basal ganglia nuclei are located deep in the cerebrum, where they surround the thalamus (Figs. 64, 65—11). Between the thalamus and these nuclei, there is a bundle of efferent and afferent nerve fibers called the internal capsule (Figs. 64, 65–12).

The basal ganglia play important roles as intermediate nuclei in the extrapyramidal system. In a complicated way, they connect the cerebrum (especially the frontal lobe), midbrain, cerebellum and spinal cord. Functionally, they contribute to the control of muscle tonus and involuntary (unconscious automatic) movements, including those that accompany voluntary movements. As a result, lesions of the basal ganglia cause abnormal muscle tonus and pathological involuntary movements (Table 5).

Table 5. BASAL GANGLIA LESIONS PRODUCING MOTOR DISTURBANCES

corpus striatum—Huntington's chorea
putamen—athetosis, dystonia
Luys' body—hemiballismus
red nucleus—rigidity (Benedikt's syndrome)
substantia nigra—Parkinson's disease

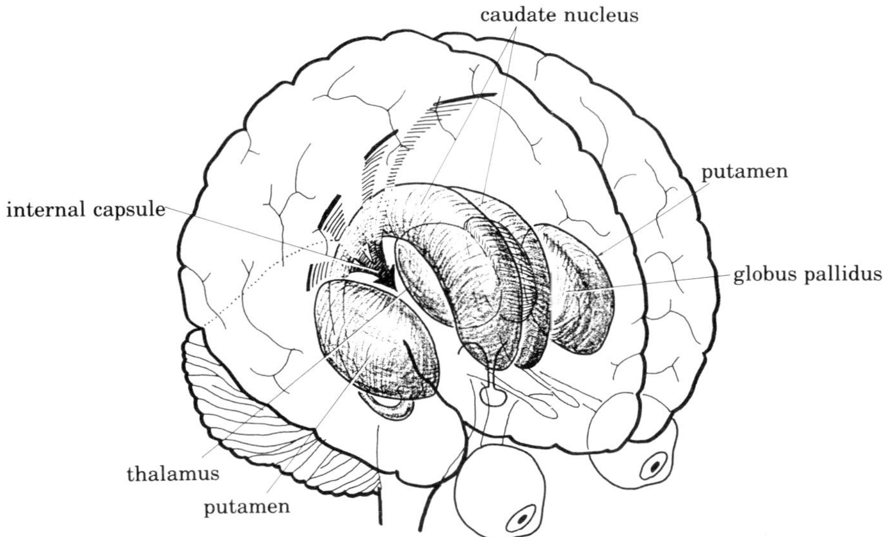

Fig. 64 The basal ganglia and thalamus.

A special neurosurgical procedure is occasionally performed within the thalamus and basal ganglia. It involves stereotaxic surgery in which the ventrolateral nuclei of the thalamus and the globus pallidus are destroyed to alleviate Parkinsonism.

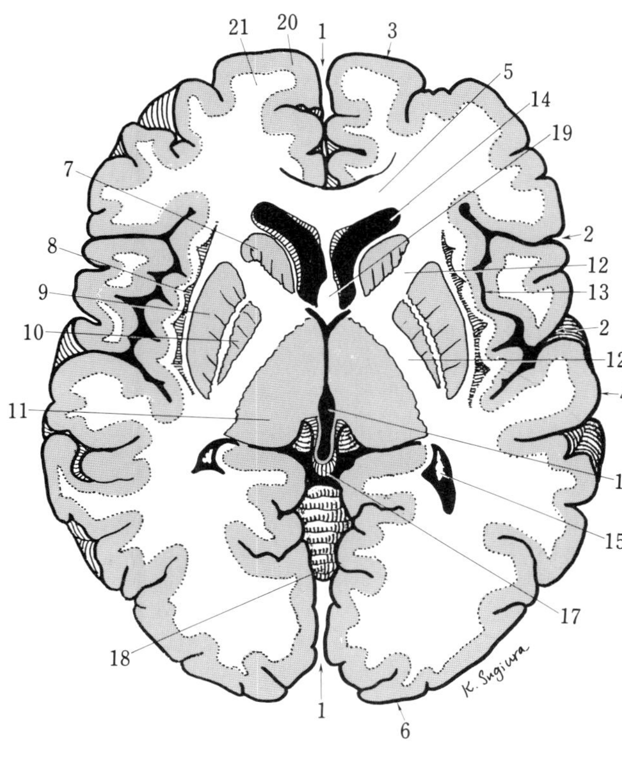

A. horizontal section of the cerebrum

B. frontal section of the cerebrum

Fig. 65 The cerebrum

1. longitudinal cerebral fissure
2. fissure of Sylvius
3. frontal lobe
4. temporal lobe
5. corpus callosum
6. occipital lobe
7. caudate nucleus
8. claustrum
9. putamen
10. globus pallidus
11. thalamus
12. internal capsule
13. insula (of Reil)
14. lateral ventricle
15. choroid plexus of lateral ventricle
16. third ventricle
17. pineal body
18. cerebellum
19. fornix
20. cerebral cortex
21. white matter of the cerebrum
22. hypothalamus
23. mammillary body
24. subthalamic nucleus
25. hippocampus

DIENCEPHALON (THALAMUS AND HYPOTHALAMUS)

The diencephalon is primarily divided into two parts, the thalamus and hypothalamus. The thalamus, which forms the lateral wall of the third ventricle, has several structures around it, including: laterally, the internal capsule; superiorly, the caudate nucleus, choroid plexus, fornix and lateral ventricle; and inferiorly, the hypothalamus (Figs, 65, 66). The two hemispheric groups of thalamic nuclei may be connected by an interthalamic adhesion, which penetrates the third ventricle. The thalamus is further divided into several nuclei, with complicated interconnections and, unfortunately, a lack of systematic nomenclature. The thalamus is divided into three nuclear groups: 1) a group receiving fibers from the reticular formation in the brain stem, which plays an important role in modulating the "alertness" of the cerebral cortex; 2) a group involved in intermediate processing of the various senses (All of the sensory intermediate nuclei, except for that of olfaction are in the thalamus. Those shown in Table 6 are aggregations of cells which process sensory information from the periphery, and relay the information to the relevant center) and 3) an evolutionary "new" group seen in advanced animals. The size of this last group in man is larger than the sum of the former two. Fibers converging here connect with association areas of the cerebral cortex and with the hypothalamus. This group functions as a processing center for higher brain functions, with outputs to many other parts of the brain.

A lesion in the thalamus produces complicated disturbances of the functions described above. The best known symptom is Dejerine-Roussy syndrome in which the patient has an extraordinary sense of numbness and intolerable pain contralateral to the lesion.

The hypothalamus is located, as the term indicates, under the thalamus and forms the antero-inferor-lateral wall of the third ventricle (Figs. 65–22, 66). It connects inferiorly with the hypophysis by way of the infundibulum. The hypothalamus is a very small part of the brain, but it has an extremely important role in the control of vegetative functions (autonomic functions). It is the "head ganglion" of the sympathetic and parasympathetic nervous systems, and also the main regulatory center for endocrine control of the hypophysis. A hypothalamic disorder may bring on an abnormality of fluid metabolism (diabetes insipidus), a disturbance of thermoregulation (hyperthermia and hypothermia), abnormal appetite (obesity and emaciation), hyper- and hypo-genitalism (pubertas praecox), and abnormal electrolyte metabolism (SIADH). All of these problems can become clinically serious conditions.

Table 6. THE RELATIONSHIP BETWEEN NUCLEI IN THE THALAMUS AND SOME SELECTED SENSES

lateral geniculate body—vision
medial geniculate body—hearing
VPM nucleus—temperature, pain, touch, taste (from the face)
VPL nucleus—temperature, pain, touch (from the body)
VL nucleus—posture and movement (cerebellar projections)
anterior nuclei—possibly small limbic projections

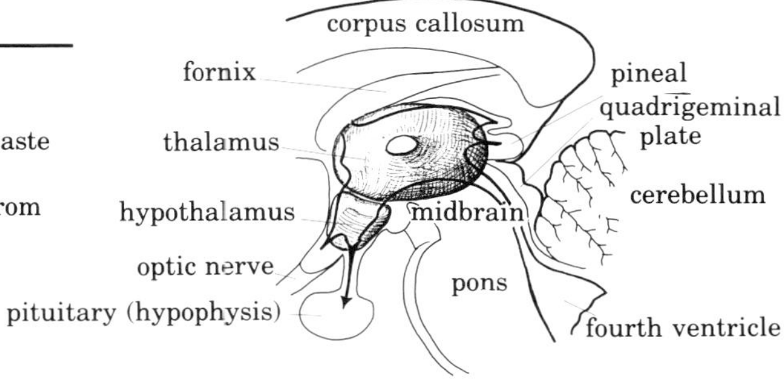

Fig. 66 The thalamus and hypothalamus.

HYPOPHYSIS AND PITUITARY GLAND

The hypophysis is extremely important for endocrine function. Located in the sella turcica where it connects with the hypothalamus by way of the infundibular stalk, it is divided into an anterior and middle lobe derived from primordia of buccal mucous membrane, and a posterior lobe which originates from nervous tissue.

The hypophysis secretes a number of hormones (Table 7) under control of releasing factors and inhibiting factors from the hypothalamus. In its posterior lobe, it stores vasopressin (antidiuretic hormone, ADH) which is manufactured by the supraoptic and paraventricular nuclei of the hypothalamus, and transported down their cells' axons (neuronsecretion) before storage in the hypophysis (Fig. 67).

Tumors originating in the hypophysis include chromophobe adenoma (mostly prolactin secretion), acidophilic adenoma (accompanying gigantism and acromegaly) and basophilic adenoma (Cushing's syndrome). Craniopharyngioma and meningioma originate from the infundibular stalk and the tuberculum sellae, respectively. The proximity of these tumors to the optic chiasm and hypothalamus helps to explain some of their symptoms (e.g., bitemporal hemianopia).

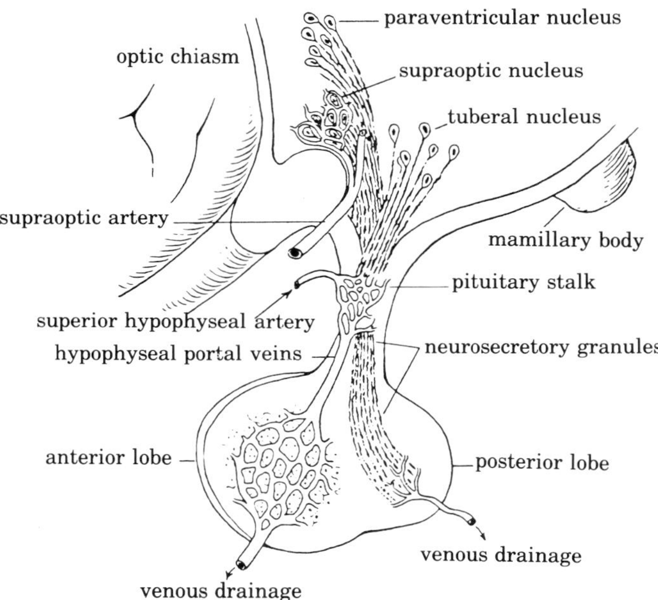

Fig. 67 Relationships between the hypothalamus and the hypophysis (after Schally).

Table 7. PITUITARY HORMONES AND THEIR CONTROL

PITUITARY HORMONES	CONTROLLING FACTORS FROM THE HYPOTHALAMUS
Anterior lobe:	
growth hormone, GH	release + inhibition
thyroid stimulating hormone, TSH	release
adrenocorticotropic hormone, ACTH	release
gonadotropic hormones, LH + FSH	release
prolactin	inhibition $>$ release
Middle lobe:	
melanocyte stimulating hormone, MSH	release + inhibition
Posterior lobe:	
antidiuretic hormone, ADH (vasopressin, oxytocin)	secreted by the hypothalamus

BRAIN STEM

Structures from the midbrain to the medulla oblongata are known as the brain stem, excluding the cerebellum (Figs. 68, 69). The midbrain penetrates the tentorial incisura, and connects to the pons, posterior to the clivus. The pons continues caudally to the medulla oblongata which emerges from the cranium through the foramen magnum to join the spinal cord in the spinal canal. The length of the brain stem is about 10 cm and its diameter is only 1–4 cm. This thin cylinder accomodates all of the information traffic between the cerebrum, cerebellum and spinal cord. Most of the cranial-nerve nuclei are located in the brain stem. Its clinical signs are summarized below. All of these characteristics are influenced by the relatively small size of the brain stem and the dense packing of its fibers and nuclei.

1. Even a lesion of small diameter (<2–3 mm) can bring on severe symptoms.
2. The cause of damage is more likely to be a hemorrhage or infarct than a tumor. Traumatic injury to the brain stem leads to particularly serious consequences.
3. The characteristic combination of symptoms caused by a brain stem lesion is paralysis of structures served by a cranial nerve on the affected side and hemiplegia on the contralateral side (alternating hemiplegia). The affected cranial nerve depends on the level of the lesion.
4. An operation near the brain stem must be performed with great caution. A lesion limited to the brain stem alone is generally inoperable.
5. Increased intracranial pressure above the tentorium forces brain tissue out the tentorial incisura. In contrast, tissue under the tentorium is forced out the foramen magnum and rarely out the tentorial incisura. Herniated brain tissue then presses on the midbrain and the medulla oblongata at the level of the tentorial incisura and the foramen magnum, respectively. Cerebral herniation at the brain stem level seriously threatens the life of the patient.

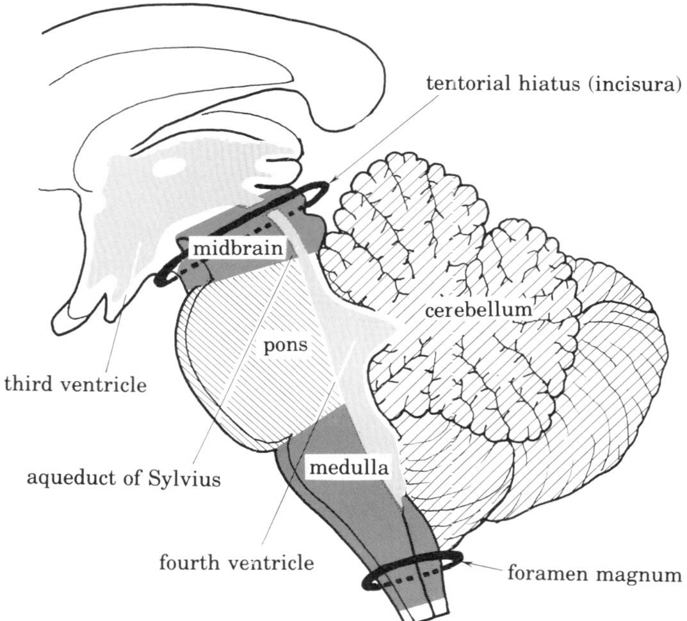

Fig. 68 The brain stem and cerebellum (sagittal section).

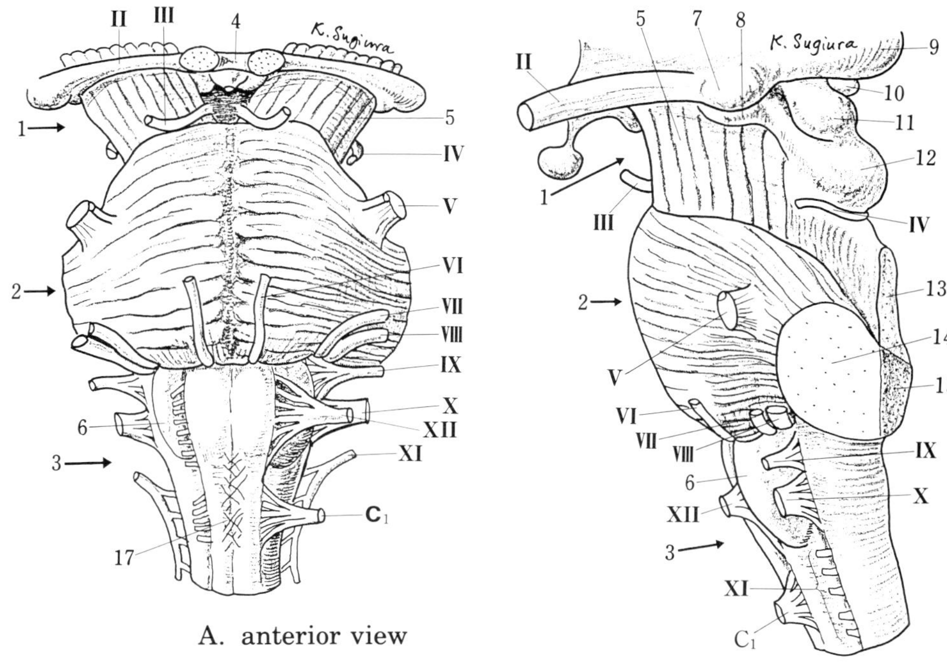

A. anterior view

B. lateral view

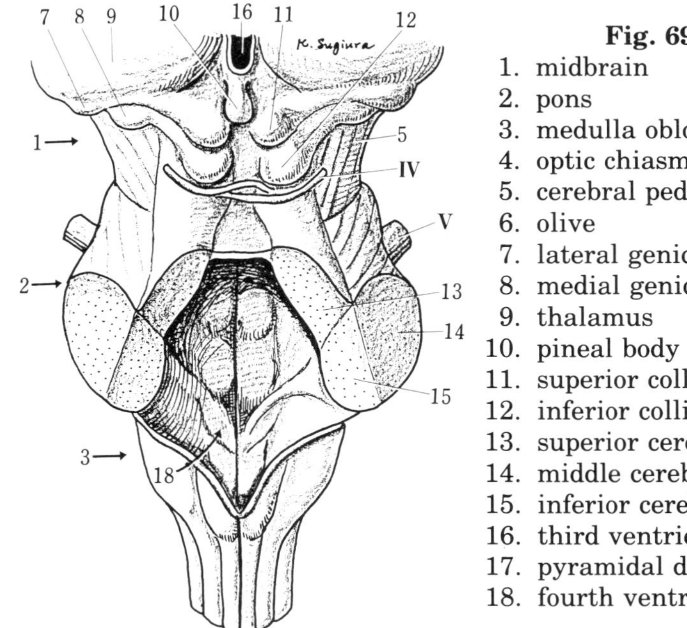

C. posterior view

Fig. 69 The brain stem.

1. midbrain
2. pons
3. medulla oblongata
4. optic chiasma
5. cerebral peduncle
6. olive
7. lateral geniculate body
8. medial geniculate body
9. thalamus
10. pineal body
11. superior colliculus } quadrigeminal plate
12. inferior colliculus } quadrigeminal plate
13. superior cerebellar peduncle
14. middle cerebellar peduncle
15. inferior cerebellar peduncle
16. third ventricle
17. pyramidal decussation
18. fourth ventricle

MIDBRAIN

The midbrain is a short part of the brain stem, 2 cm long, lying between the diencephalon and the pons. It is bordered anteriorly by the cerebral peduncle (69–5) and posteriorly by the quadrigeminal plate (69–11, 12).

The cerebral peduncle (69–5, 70–11), contains fibers of the pyramidal tract projecting from the posterior limb of the internal capsule. Deep to the peduncle lies the substantia nigra (70–12), a prominent nucleus of the extrapyramidal system, which is a well-known lesion site in Parkinsonism. The dorsal part of the midbrain, ventral to the cerebral aqueduct (70–1), is called the tegmentum. It includes a large number of connecting fibers coursing up and down the brain stem and several nuclei including the red, oculomotor and trochlear nuclei and the mesencephalic nucleus of the trigeminal nerve. The red nucleus (70–10), another prominent component of the extrapyramidal system, is known to be a lesion site in Benedikt's syndrome (70–A) whose signs include abnormal muscle tone and involuntary movement. The oculomotor nucleus (70–III) is located just anterior to the cerebral aqueduct. Its fibers (oculomotor nerve) penetrate the tegmentum and proceed out of the midbrain medially to the cerebral peduncle (70–III). As a result, hemorrhage in the cerebral peduncle can produce contralateral hemiplegia and, simultaneously, ipsilateral paralysis of structures supplied by the oculomotor nerve. This combination is known as Weber's syndrome (70–A).

There are four mounds on the dorsal surface of the quadrigeminal plate. They comprise two pairs of colliculi (69–11, 12). The superior pair contain nuclei controlling eye reflexes, gaze functions and pupillary reflexes. Damage to this area produces Parinaud's syndrome and Argyll Robertson's syndrome, with symptoms in both eyes and pupils. The inferior colliculi are intermediate processing stations for hearing.

An important clinical fact is that the midbrain penetrates the tentorial incisura. If treatment for increased pressure above the tentorium is delayed, parts of the temporal lobe are usually forced out the tentorial incisura, where they press on the midbrain. This is called tentorial herniation. By damaging the reticular formation behind the midbrain, it causes decerebrate rigidity. This motor symptom is important together with anisocoria (with paralysis of structures supplied by the oculomotor nerve) for indicating tentorial herniation.

PONS

The pons lies between the midbrain and the medulla oblongata. The posterior wall of the pons forms the base of the fourth ventricle (Fig. 68), behind which the cerebellum is located. The pons and the cerebellum are connected by the middle cerebellar peduncle (69–14, 70–25). The ventral surface of the pons, called the basilar part, contains transverse pontine fibers, which link the cerebral cortex with the cerebellum via pontine nuclei. The pyramidal tract (70–23), which courses through the basilar part, is an extension of the cerebral peduncle. Its fibers project to the medulla, passing perpendicularly through the transverse pontine fibers.

The pontine tegmentum in the dorsal part of the pons is comprised of connecting fibers and several nuclei of cranial nerves, including: 1) the motor nucleus of the trigeminal nerve and the pontine nucleus (98–2, 4), 2) the abducens nucleus (70–VI) and its accessory nucleus (center for conjugate gaze), 3) the facial nucleus (70–VII) and 4) the vestibular and cochlear nuclei (98–6, 7).

Syndromes produced by a lesion in the pons include:

1. The Millard-Gubler syndrome (70–B)
   Facial palsy on the affected side with or without an abducens paralysis on the affected side and hemiplegia on the contralateral side.

2. The Foville syndrome (70–B)
   Paralysis of horizontal gaze and abducens paralysis, with or without facial palsy on the affected side, with or without contralateral hemiplegia.
3. The Locked-in syndrome
4. The cerebello-pontine angle syndrome

These syndromes have particular significance because their various combinations rarely occur after lesions of other brain regions.

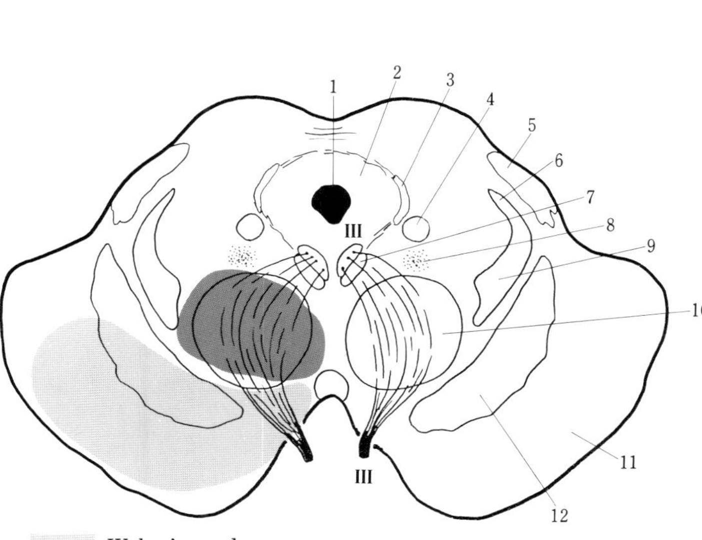

A. midbrain and common positions of lesions

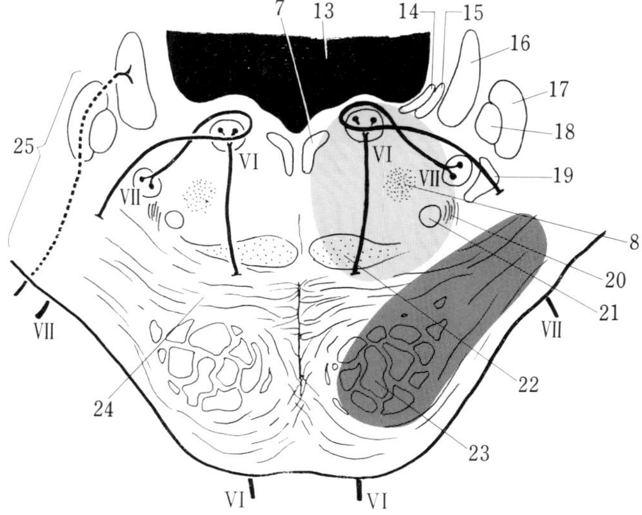

B. pons and common positions of lesions

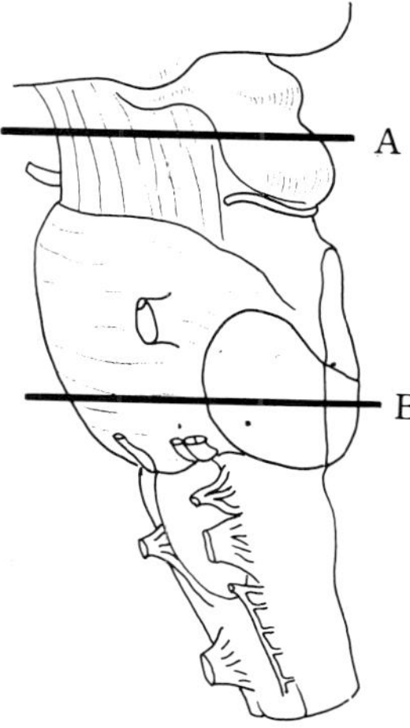

Fig. 70 Horizontal sections of the brain stem.

1. cerebral aqueduct
2. central gray substance
3. mesencephalic nucleus of the trigeminal nerve
4. bulbothalamic tract
5. brachium of the inferior colliculus
6. lateral spinothalamic tract
7. medial longitudinal fasciculus
8. central tegmental tract
9. medial lemniscus
10. red nucleus
11. cerebral peduncle (pyramidal tract)
12. substantia nigra
13. fourth ventricle
14. superior salivary nucleus
15. lacrimal nucleus
16. superior vestibular nucleus
17. spinal trigeminal tract
18. spinal trigeminal nucleus
19. rubrospinal tract
20. lateral lemniscus
21. superior olivary nucleus
22. trapezoid body of the medial lemniscus
23. pyramidal tract
24. transverse pontine fibers
25. middle cerebellar peduncle

MEDULLA OBLONGATA

The medulla oblongata is the most caudal part of the brain stem. It extends below the pons, through the foramen magnum, to connect with the spinal cord. The medulla has centers for respiration, swallowing, blood circulation and vomiting. These functions are essential for life. Consequently, cerebellar (tonsillar) herniation is fatal, because these centers are then damaged by ptosis of the cerebellar tonsils.

The pyramidal tract (71–10) is located medio-ventrally in the medulla. Caudally, it interdigitates at the midline (pyramidal decussation 69–17) and continues on in the lateral funiculus of the spinal cord (75–15). The medulla is not only comprised of several nerve pathways, but also contains nuclei of the IXth, Xth, XIth and XIIth cranial nerves, the nucleus of the trigeminal nerve (71–7), and the olivary nuclei (71–9; note the important connections with the cerebellum), and the cuneate and gracile nuclei. Syndromes (none of which are necessarily fatal) caused by lesions of the medulla include: Jackson's syndrome*, Wallenberg's syndrome** and bulbar palsy*** (Fig. 71).

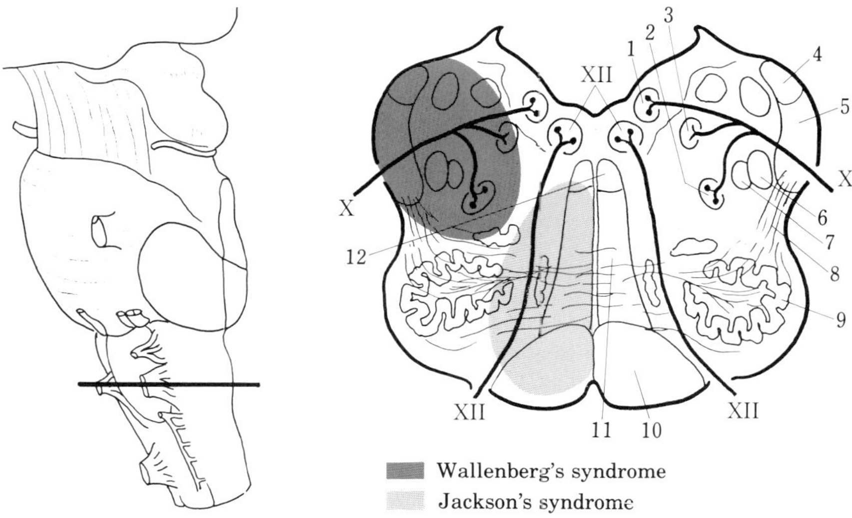

Fig. 71 A section at the medullary level.

1. dorsal nucleus of the vagus nerve
2. nucleus ambiguus
3. solitary nucleus
4. spinocerebellar tract
5. inferior cerebellar peduncle
6. spinal tract of the trigeminal nerve
7. spinal nucleus of trigeminal nerve
8. olivary-cerebellar tract
9. inferior olivary nucleus
10. pyramid (tract)
11. medial lemniscus
12. medial longitudinal fasciculus

---

* A type of alternating hemiplegia resulting from a pyramidal tract lesion. Hypoglossal nerve paralysis on the affected side and contralateral side hemiplegia.

** Caused by a lateral medulla lesion. Most cases involve thrombosis within the posterior inferior cerebellar or vertebral arteries. On the affected side, this produces: 1) disturbance of the trigeminal nerve, 2) Horner's syndrome, 3) ataxia and 4) bulbar palsy. On the contralateral side occasionally, 5) a hemihypoesthesia.

***Results from IXth through XIIth cranial nerve damage within the medulla, leading to a combination of disorders involving hoarseness, dysphagia and dysarthria.

CEREBELLUM

The cerebellum is located in the posterior cranial fossa, posterior to the pons and to the medulla. Its superior and lateral surfaces are covered by the tentorium cerebelli upon which the cerebrum is supported. The cerebellum is divided into a vermis, which is located medially, and a left and right hemisphere (72–2).

The cell bodies of cerebellar neurons are found in the cerebellar cortex and four deep structures, the dentate, fastigial, emboliform and globose nuclei. Fiber connections between the cerebellum and other parts of the brain are by way of three pairs of cerebellar peduncles. These are the superior cerebellar peduncle (72–4), the middle cerebellar peduncle (72–6) and the inferior cerebellar peduncle (72–5). They have connections with the midbrain, the pons and the medulla, respectively.

The peduncles carry information (including visual and auditory) to the cerebellum and return a cerebellar-processed version to brain regions that supplied the original information. Thus, the cerebellum, acting subconsciously, functions as a coordinating center, particularly for the motor system. The main function of the cerebellum is to judge the appropriateness of body movements and to point out corrections if errors have occurred. Primary motor cortex commands the hands and feet to move voluntarily, but the cerebellum is needed to ensure that these movements are executed smoothly and correctly.

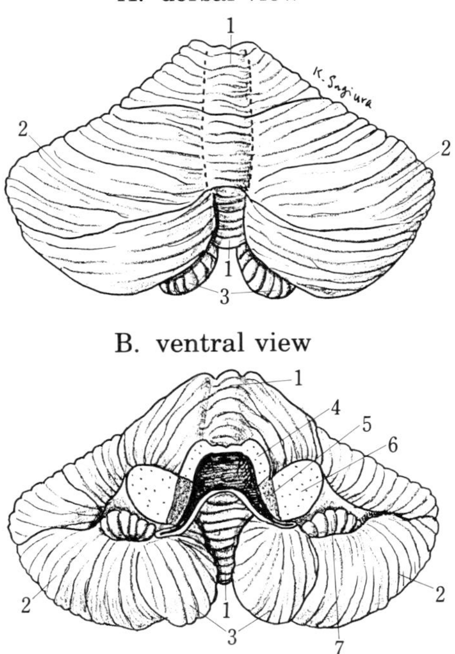

Fig. 72 The cerebellum.
1. vermis
2. cerebellar hemisphere
3. tonsils
4. superior cerebellar peduncle
5. inferior cerebellar peduncle
6. middle cerebellar peduncle
7. flocculus

Symptoms of cerebellar disorders include:

1. Ataxic gait: The patient is prone to stagger and stumble even when using a wide-based gait. In the case of an unilateral hemispheric disorder, the motor deficit is more on the affected side.
2. Truncal ataxia: This follows damage to the vermis, with difficulty encountered in keeping the body upright in both standing and sitting postures.
3. Dysmetria: This is checked by finger-to-finger, finger-to-nose and heel-to-knee tests. If the cerebellum is damaged, movements directed toward a target cannot be executed smoothly, and are often in the wrong direction (Fig. 73).
4. Adiadochokinesia: This disorder is revealed by rhythmically swinging both hands backwards and forwards. There is an impaired ability to start a movement in the reverse direction.
5. Dysarthria: Without appropriate cerebellar control of the muscles of the tongue and mouth, the patient can not speak smoothly. Their speech is inarticulate, even without aphasia.
6. Hypotonia: The patient exhibits a lower-than-normal tone while their limbs are being flexed and extended by the examiner. Tendon-jerk reflexs are also depressed in many cases.
7. Intention tremor: This differs from tremor at rest seen in Parkinson patients. Rather, during an active goal-directed movement (e.g., the finger-to-nose test), the tremor becomes larger as the finger approaches the nose (73–B).
8. Nystagmus: This involuntary movement of the eyes occurs after damage to any of the connections between the vestibular nucleus, the cerebellum and the eye-movement system. Nystagmus is classified by its timing (gazing, changing head position), features (horizontal, rotating, perpendicular) and direction of movement. Additionally, cerebellar damage can lead to ataxic nystagmus, a form of dysmetria in which the eyes exhibit movement at rest and cannot track a moving object.

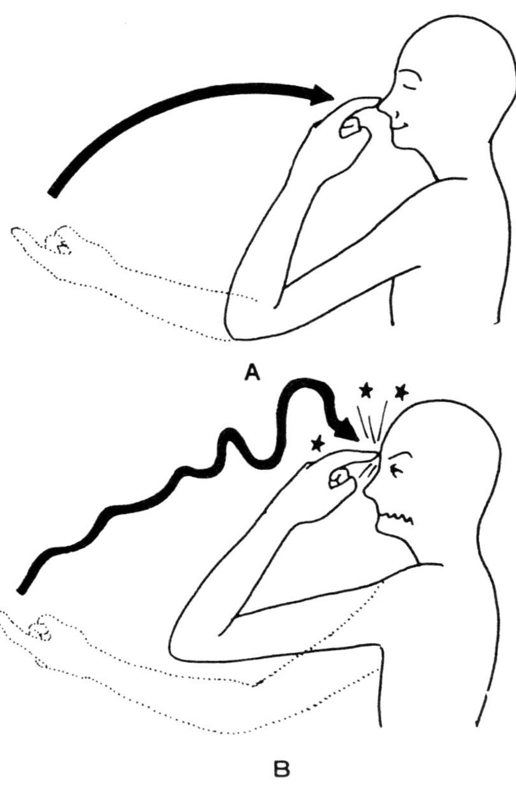

Fig. 73 Dysmetria and intention tremor.

A normal subject (A) can point to their nose quite accurately. If cerebellar ataxia is evident (B), the patient displays progressively more tremor as the hand approaches the target (intention tremor). Finally, the movement is elaborated in the wrong direction.

SPINAL CORD

The spinal cord is housed within the bony spinal column where it is protected from external forces. In adults, the conus medullaris, at the caudal end of the spinal cord, is at the level of the first lumbar vertebra. Below this level, all that remains is the cauda equina (Fig. 76). The length of the spinal cord and of the spinal column is almost the same in the embryo until the third month. Afterwards, the vertebrae grow faster than the spinal cord, such that the cord becomes suspended upwards, with its caudal end as high as the third lumbar vertebra in a newborn child. The difference in level, between infants and adults, of the caudal end of the spinal cord should be recognized before proceeding with a lumbar puncture.

The spinal cord is covered by the same three meningeal coverings seen in the brain. These are: the outermost dura mater, the arachnoid (including cerebrospinal fluid) and the pia mater, which tightly invests the cord. In the cranium, the dura mater consists of both periosteum and the dura mater itself. Conversely, in the spinal cord, the dura mater exists separate from the periosteum. As a result, a space, called the epidural cavity (74–2), is found between the dura mater and the periosteum and ends at the foramen magnum. Epidural anesthesia is safer than spinal anesthesia because the local anesthetic does not diffuse into the cranium.

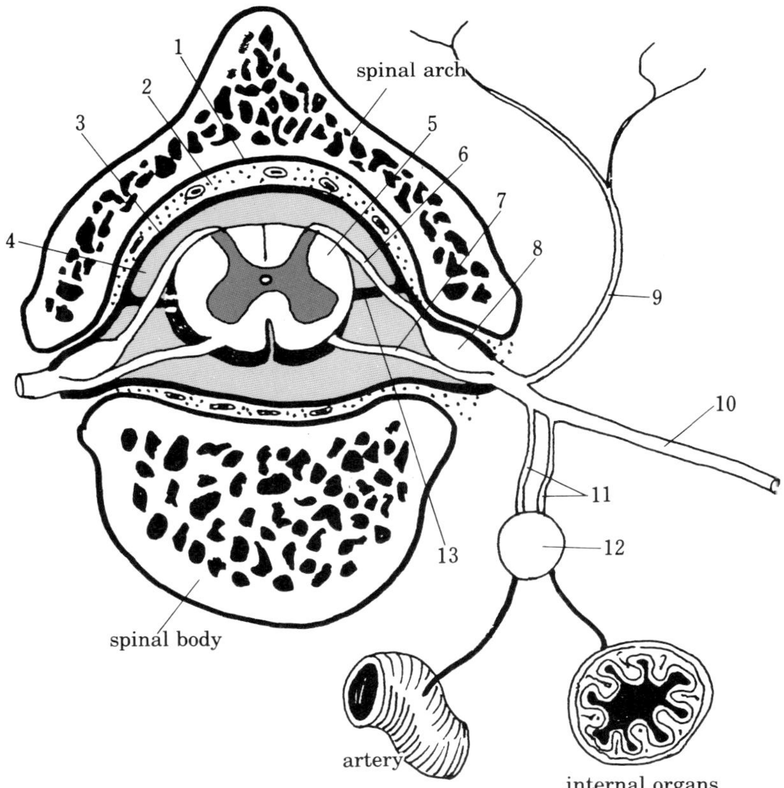

Fig. 74 The spinal cord and spinal nerves.

1. periosteum
2. epidural cavity
3. dura mater and arachnoid
4. subarachnoid space
5. spinal cord
6. dorsal root
7. ventral root
8. spinal ganglion
9. posterior ramus
10. anterior ramus
11. sympathetic communicans
12. sympathetic trunk ganglion
13. dentate ligament

In the spinal cord, the grey matter, composed of nerve cell bodies, is located internal to the white matter, which is composed of nerve fibers. This arrangement is the reverse of that seen in the brain (Fig. 75). It is essential to grasp the gross architectural features of the cord, including its anterior, lateral and posterior horns, and the anterior, lateral and posterior funiculi.

The anterior horn (75–1) contains cell bodies controlling movement. They extend to the anterior root. Descending fibers which terminate on or near these cells include some from the pyramidal tract (75–15) which descends all the way from the frontal lobe. The lateral horn (75–2) contains sympathetic nerve cells whose fibers emerge from the spinal cord as part of the anterior root. The nerve cells contained in the posterior horn (75–3) have a sensory function. Sensory input concerning temperature and pain enter into spinal cord via the posterior root (75–8), and then interacts with cells in the posterior horn.

Among the various tracts coursing up and down in the white matter, the most clinically distinguishable ones include the pain-temperature pathway (spinothalamic tract) (75–16), the lateral corticospinal tract (75–15) (both running in the lateral funiculus) and the tactile-kinesthetic (dorsal-column) pathway which ascends through the posterior funiculus (fasciculus cuneatus, 75–14, and fasciculus gracilis 75–13). These pathways are described later.

There are 31 pairs of spinal nerves exiting from the spinal cord. A spinal nerve (75–10) consists of an anterior root, composed of efferent (motor) fibers, and a posterior root, composed of afferent (sensory) fibers. Thus, the spinal cord can be divided into segments, each of which has an anterior and a posterior root. A single segment is shown in Fig.75. The cervical cord (C), thoracic cord (T or Th), lumbar cord (L) and sacral cord (S) is each composed of several spinal segments, and are anatomically related to their corresponding vertebrae. Nerves from these regions are called the cervical, thoracic, lumbar and sacral nerves, respectively. Due to the abovementioned difference in the growth rate of the spinal cord and spinal column, most spinal segments are at a higher level than their corresponding vertebrae. The lower the segment, the longer the distance its root must travel to emerge from the spinal canal. As shown in Figure 76, the levels are quite different for each spinal segment, vertebral body and spinal process. If this is not understood, errors are likely to occur when localizing spinal lesions during an examination or operation.

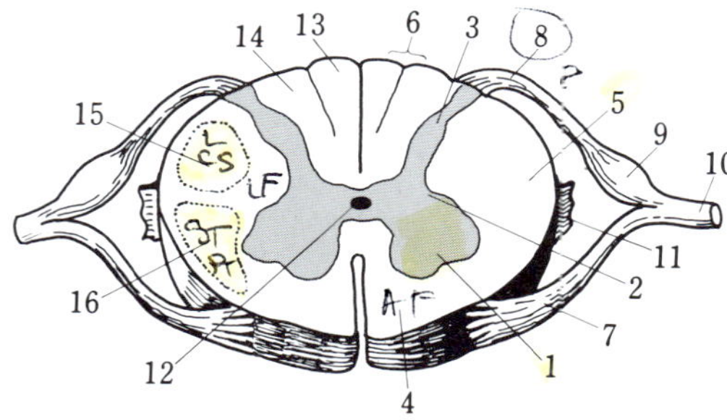

Fig. 75 A single spinal segment.

1. anterior horn
2. lateral horn
3. posterior horn
4. anterior funiculus
5. lateral funiculus
6. posterior funiculus
7. anterior root
8. posterior root
9. spinal ganglion
10. spinal nerve
11. dentate ligament
12. central canal
13. fasciculus gracilis
14. fasciculus cuneatus
15. pyramidal tract
16. spinothalamic tract

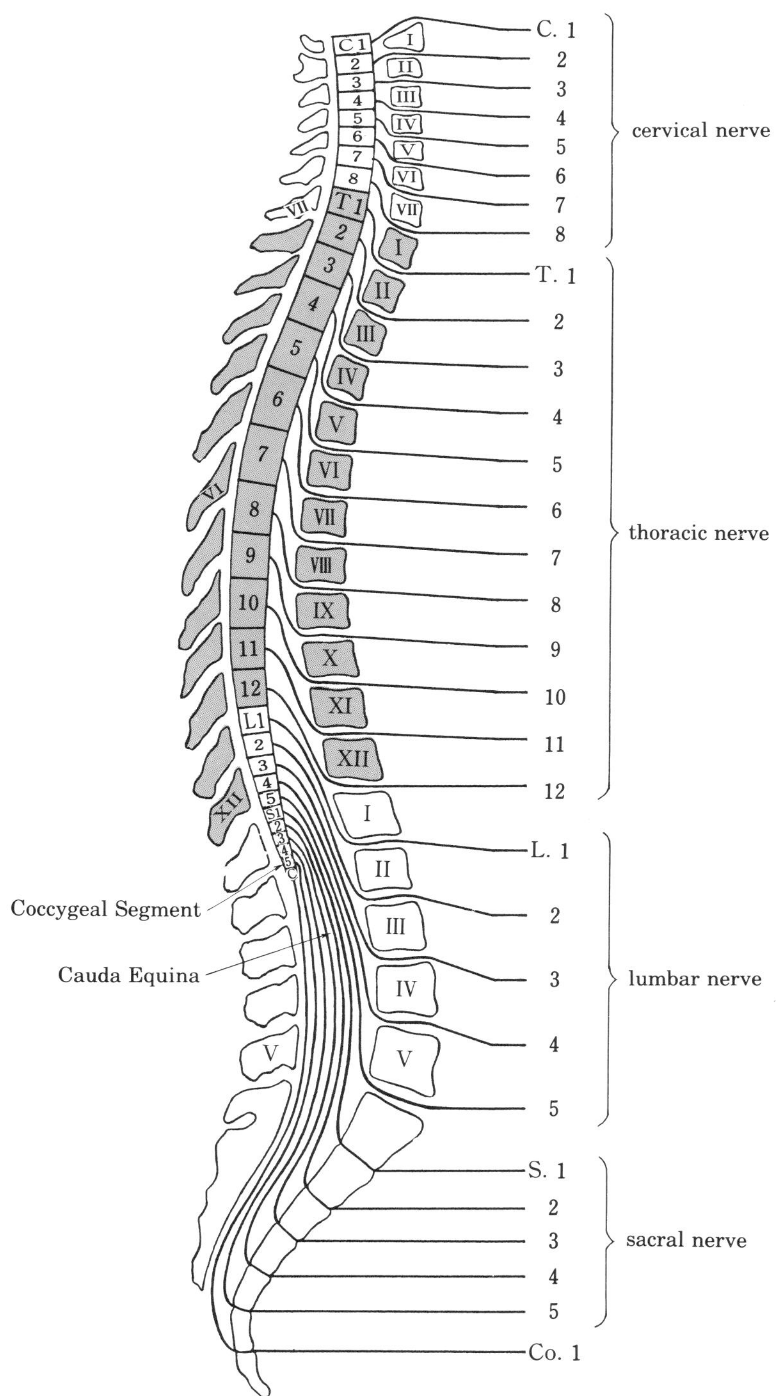

Fig. 76 The spinal vertebrae, spinal cord and spinal nerves.
Note the different levels of the vertebral bodies, their spinous processes and their corresponding spinal segments. Caudally, the spinal cord tapers to end at the first lumbar vertebra, with the cauda equina extending below.

A belt-like skin area innervated by the posterior root of each single spinal nerve is called a dermatome (Fig. 77). This segmental distribution is very important when deciding on the level of a lesion in the spinal cord. Representative symptoms of spinal damage include: 1) paraplegia or quadriplegia - with differences depending on the specific sites of the lesion, 2) vesicorectal disturbances and 3) Brown-Sequard syndrome. A combination of 1 and 2 caused by cervical cord damage is particularly debilitating. The patient cannot move the arms and legs at all, is incontinent and breathes with difficulty. Furthermore, they clearly realize these hardships, because consciousness is never disturbed. Those involved in the treatment of, or operations for, spinal disorders should bear in mind that damage to this narrow region, of just a finger's breadth, can have shattering consequences. Operations performed on the cord and column include laminectomy (to remove tumors), anterior fusion (to stabilize the spine), and antero-lateral cordotomy to selectively destroy a part of the spinal cord (to reduce pain).

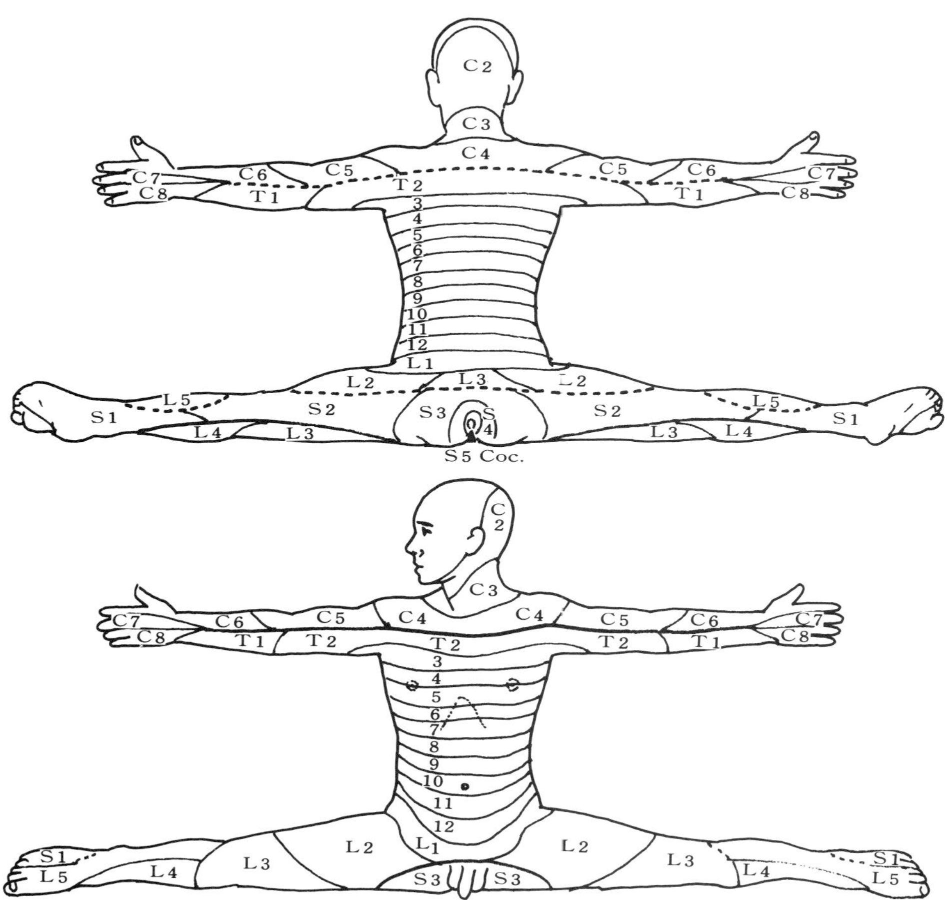

Fig. 77 The segmental distribution of spinal sensory nerves (after Haymaker and Woodhall).

Locations to be learned include:

C2:	back of the head	T4:	areola mammae
C3:	neck	T10:	navel
C4:	shoulder	L2,3+S2:	thigh
C5–T2:	upper extremity	L4,5+S1:	leg
		below S3:	groin

COMPUTERIZED TOMOGRAPHY OF THE HEAD

Computerized tomography of the head (abbreviation, CT) was put into practical use in 1973 by Hounsfield in England. He revolutionized the examination of all body structures, including the brain. Computerized tomography involves: X-ray radiation of pin-point size passing through the body and being detected, calculation of the absorption per division (pixel) of arbitrary body sections and finally, an output display on a TV screen (Figs. 78, 79).

Since radiation absorption differs from tissue to tissue (Fig. 80), high and low absorption areas are seen as white and black, respectively, in a scanning image adjusted for human recognition. Recent technology has allowed for greater distinction between white (fibers) and grey matter (cortex and nuclei) and for the detection of brain edema. A hematoma is clearly visible because it exhibits very high (white) absorption.

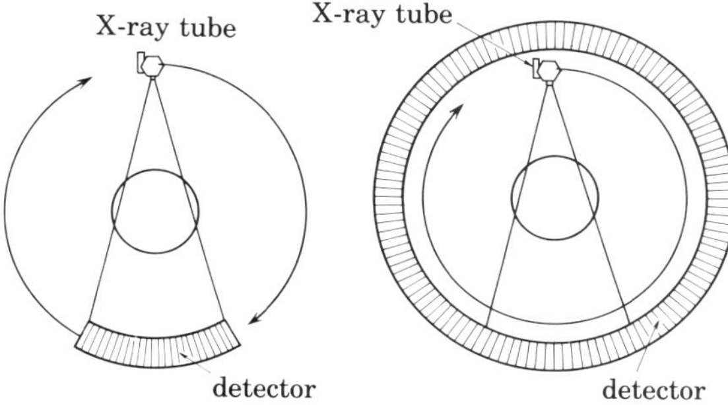

Fig. 78 The principles of computerized tomography.

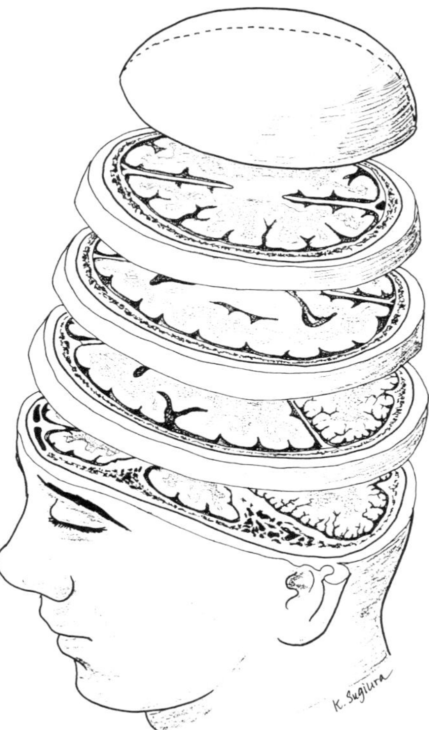

A CT scan after injection of contrast media (including iodine) should show no change in normal parts of the brain, because of the blood brain barrier. However, it will show high absorption in areas rich in blood or with an impaired or absent blood-brain barrier (e.g. brain tumors, infarcts, aneurysms and arteriovenous malformations). This property is called contrast enhancement. It greatly helps in the examination of various tumors (Fig. 81).

Fig. 79 A diagram showing the application of computerized tomography.

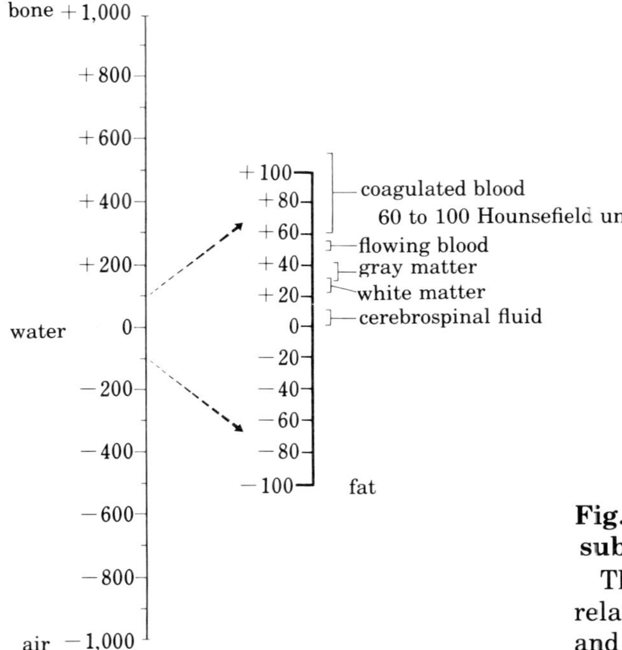

Fig. 80 Absorption of different substances (Hounsefield units).
The absorption values are shown in relation to bone (+1000), air (−1000) and water (spinal fluid) (0).

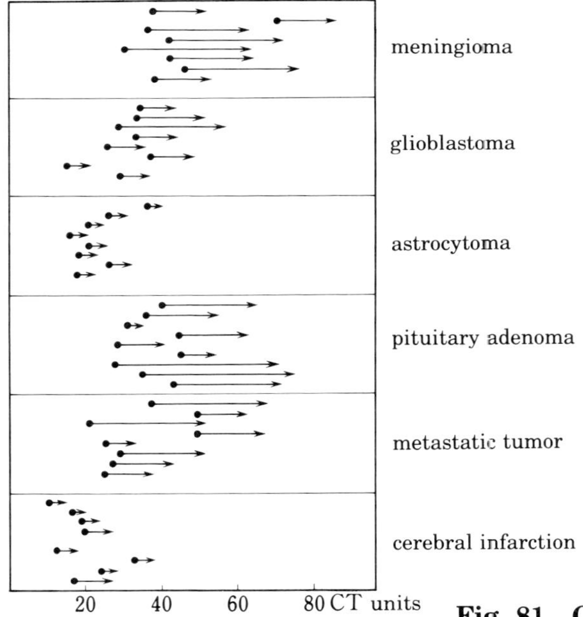

Fig. 81 Contrast enhancement and the change of absorption (by Lange and colleagues).

When examining a CT scan, the angle of section must be considered. Scanning is generally done in planes parallel to a line connecting the lateral canthus and the external acoustic meatus (82–B). However, the actual angle is changeable depending on available equipment and other technical issues. Small differences in the angle of section make large differences in the viewed images (Fig. 82). To prevent misinterpretations, it is necessary to read images three-dimensionally with recognition of: 1) intracranial structures, such as ventricles and cisterns, 2) bony structures (orbital cavity, sella turcica, sphenoidal wing, and the petrosal part of temporal bone) and 3) the lateral border of the head.

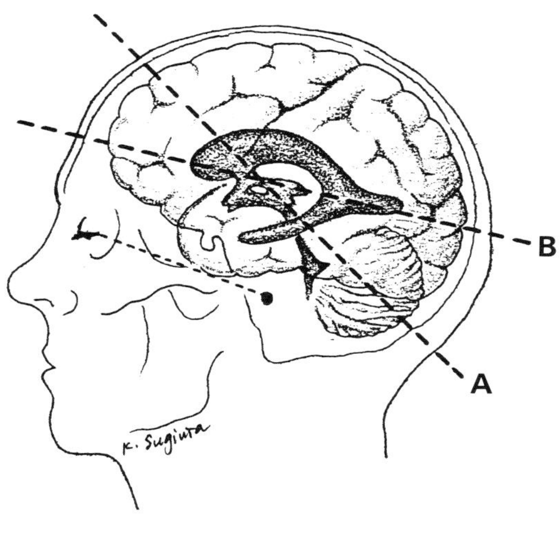

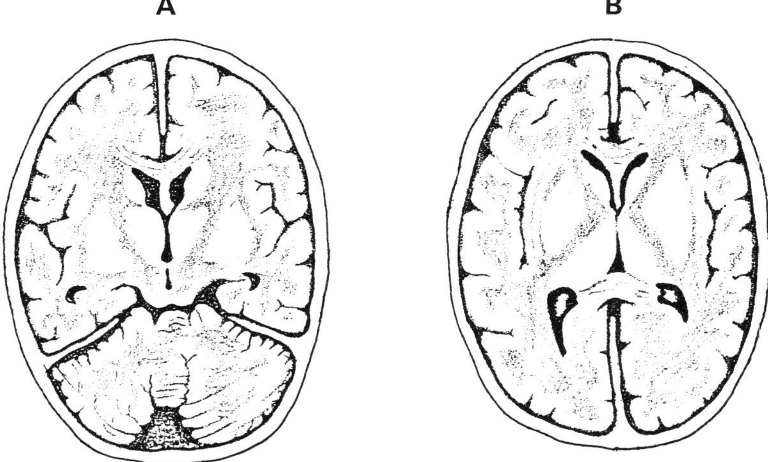

Fig. 82 Effects of changing the plane of section on the CT scan.

NORMAL CT SCANS (Figs. 83–90)

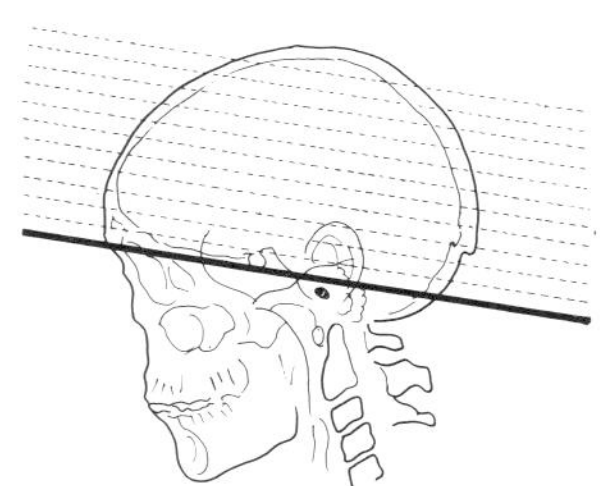

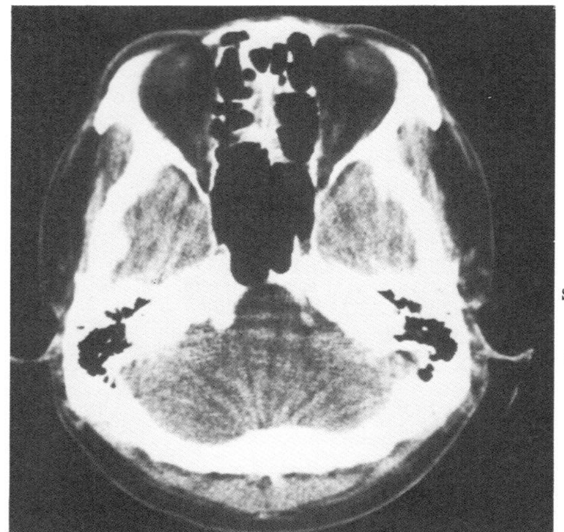

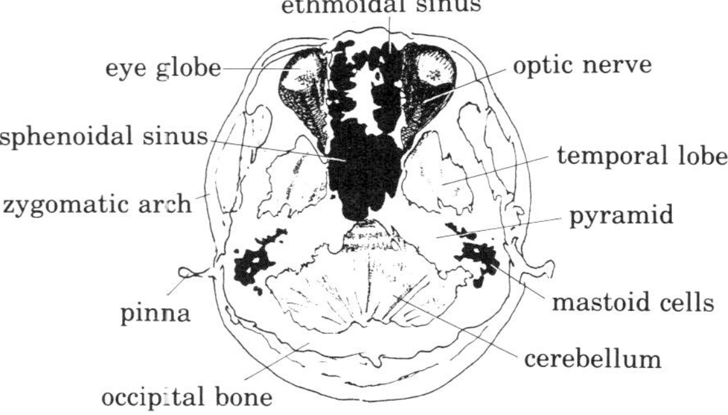

Fig. 83

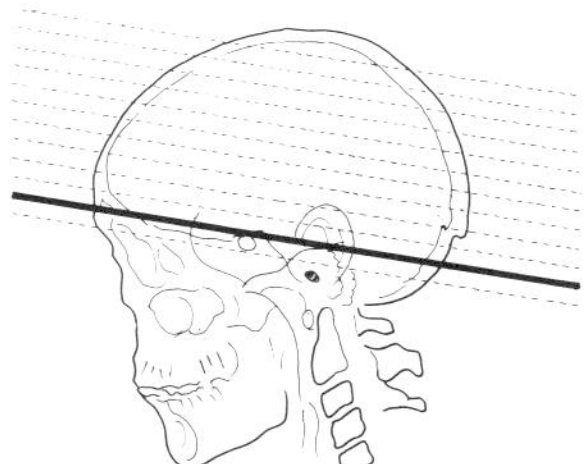

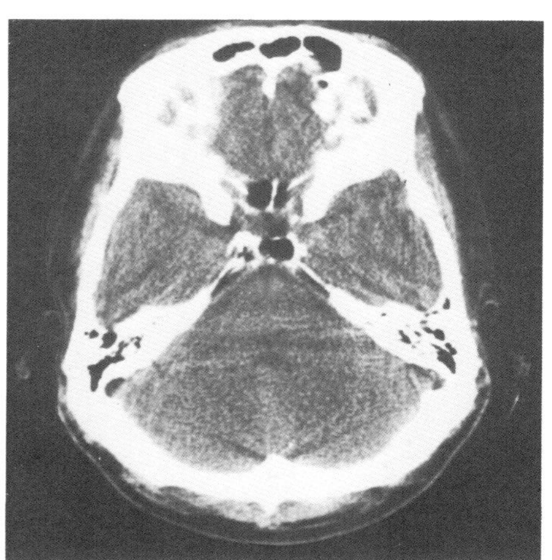

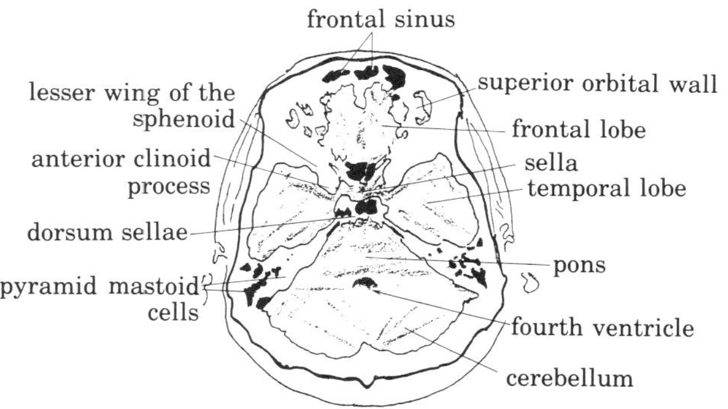

Fig. 84

frontal bone
frontal lobe
sylvian fissure
sphenoidal ridge
chiasmatic cistern
interpeduncular cistern
temporal horn
crural cistern
lateral ventricle
temporal lobe
ambient cistern
midbrain
cerebellum

Fig. 85

frontal bone
frontal lobe
frontal horn
third ventricle
hypothalamus
sylvian fissure
quadrigeminal plate
insula
temporal lobe
quadrigeminal cistern
cerebellum
occipital lobe

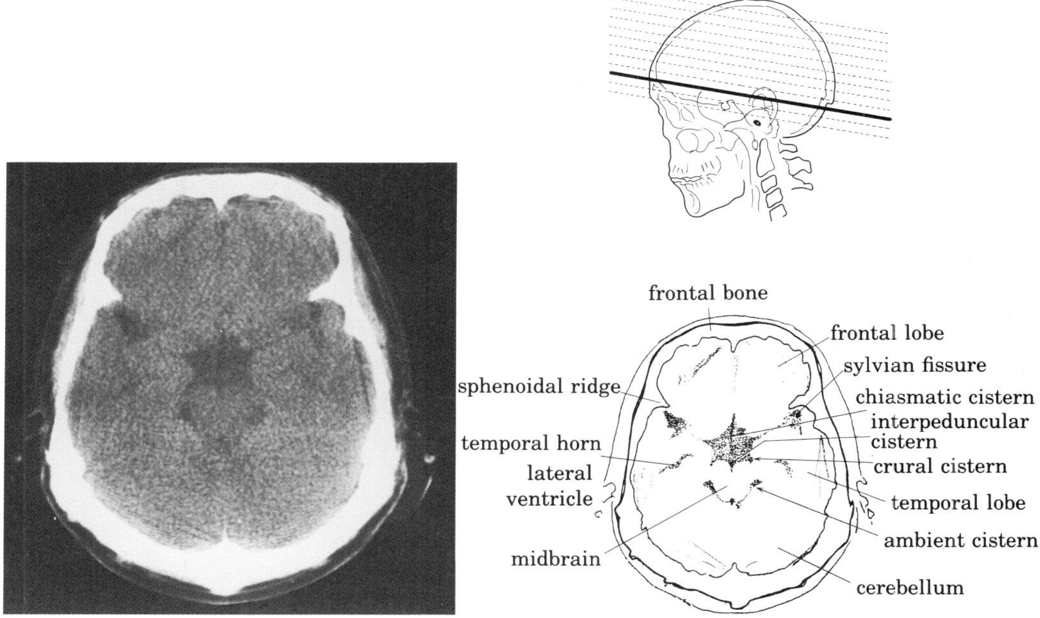

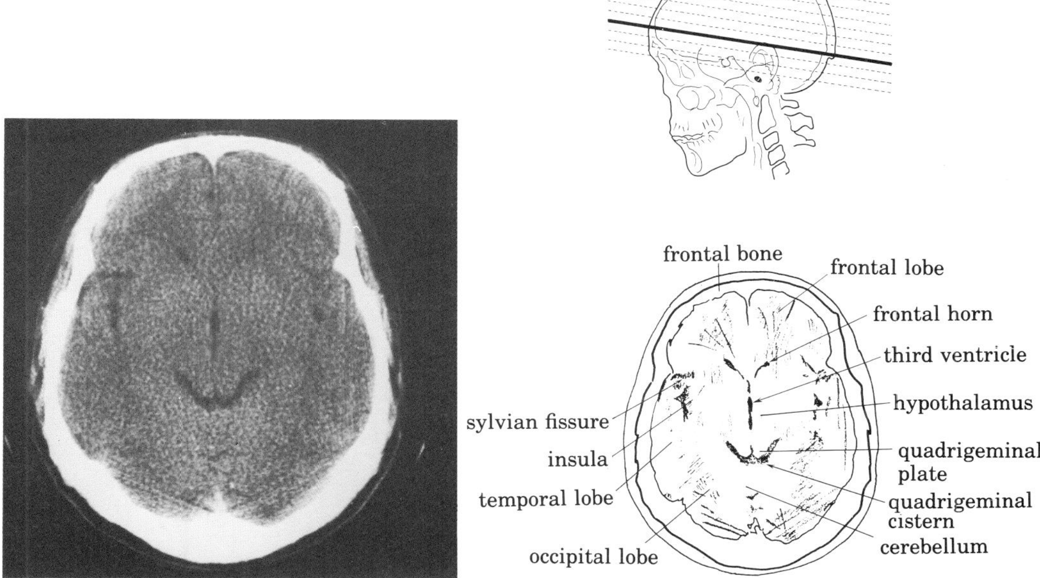

Fig. 86

frontal bone
frontal lobe
corpus callosum
septum pellicidum
frontal horn
caudate nucleus (head)
foramen of
Monro
internal capsule
anterior limb
insula
lenticular nucleus
temporal lobe
internal capsule
posterior limb
third ventricle
thalamus
pineal
occipital lobe
cerebellar vermis

Fig. 87

interhemispheric fissure
frontal lobe
caudate nucleus
lenticular
nucleus
temporal lobe
internal capsule,
posterior limb
thalamus
trigone of the
lateral ventricle
calcified choroid
plexus
occipital lobe

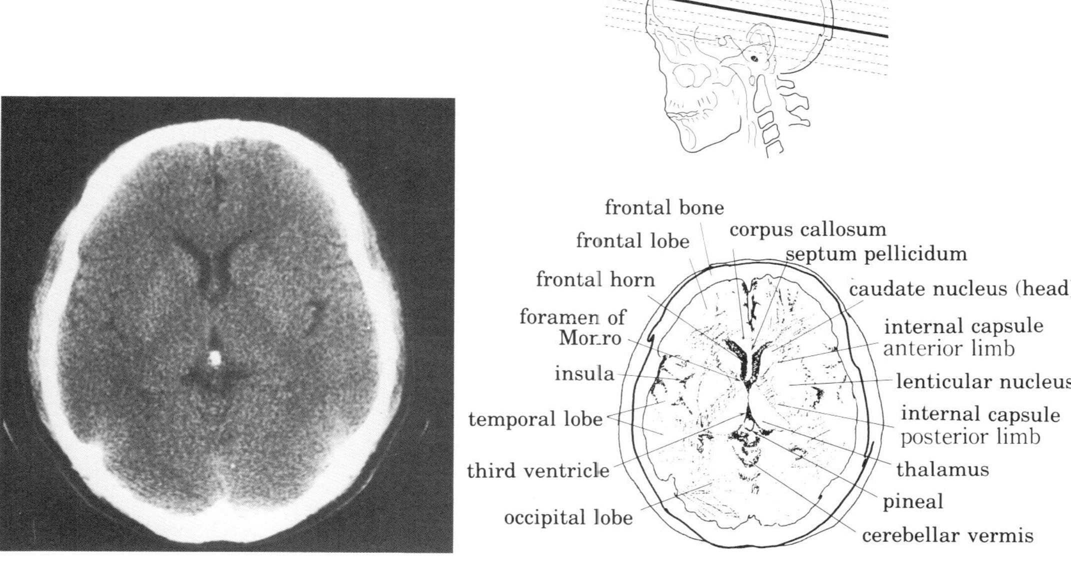

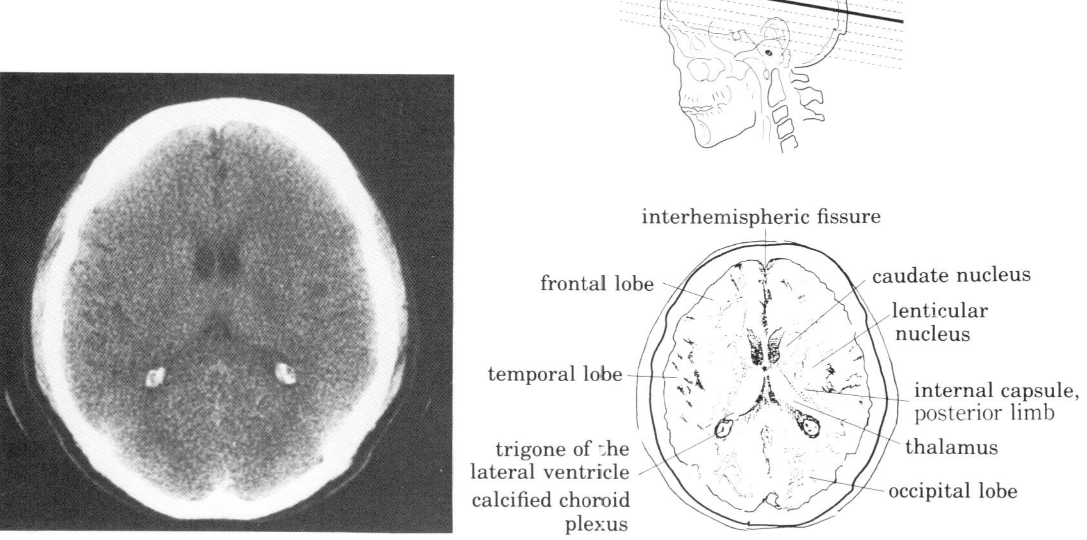

Fig. 88

frontal lobe
corpus callosum
caudate
nucleus (body)
corona radiata
body of the
lateral ventricle
parietal lobe
falx cerebri
occipital lobe
interhemispheric
fissure

Fig. 89

frontal lobe
sulci
parietal lobe
falx cerebri
centrum
semiovale
interhemispheric
fissure
occipital lobe

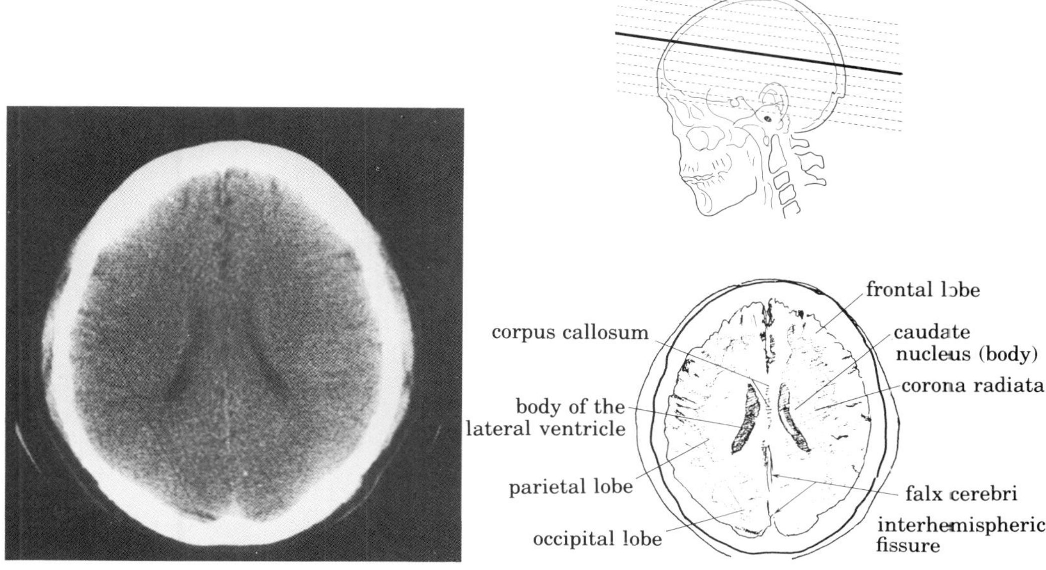

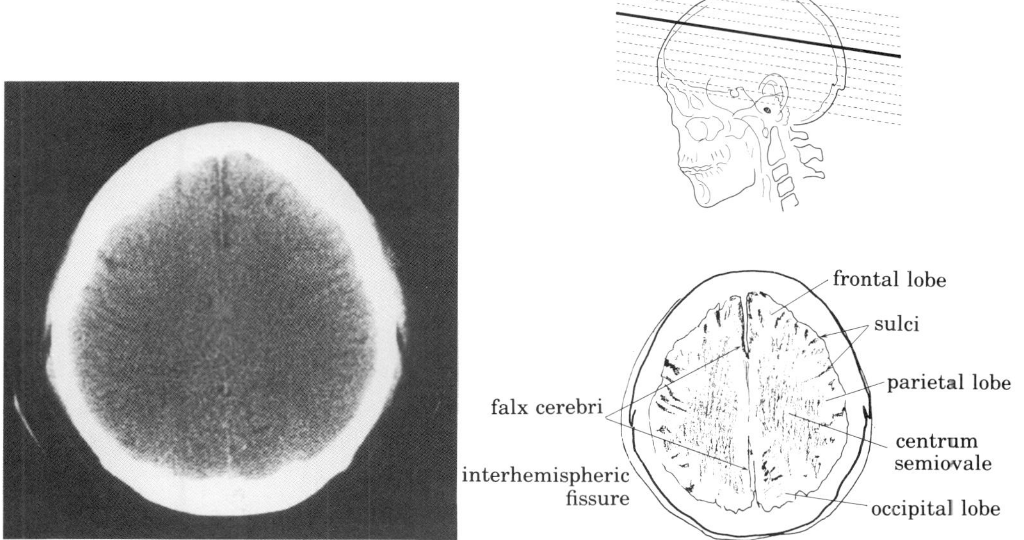

Fig. 90

Case 11: 57 year old male; hypertensive intracerebral hematoma

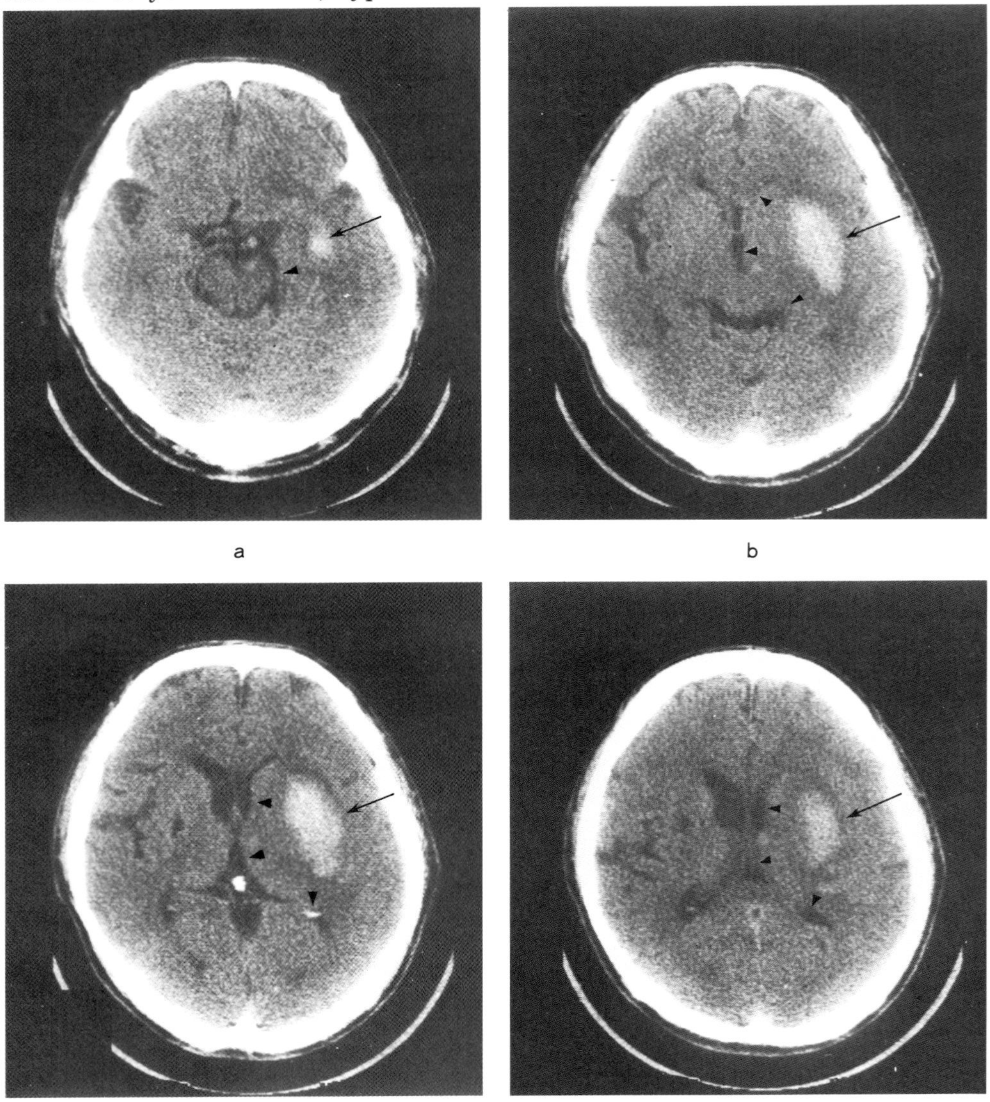

a

b

c

d

Fig. 91

Three days prior to examination, the patient kept falling and staggering and was unable to walk. He kept resting, but muscle weakness persisted on the left side. Upon admission, his blood pressure was 170/80 mm Hg. He was conscious, with paresis clearly evident on the left side of his body.

CT scanning revealed a mass with high absorption centered in the right putamen, consistent with an acute hematoma (←), with low absorption around it due to edema. A slight dislocation and deformity of the ventricles was also seen (◀).

Case 12: 51 year old male; metastatic tumor

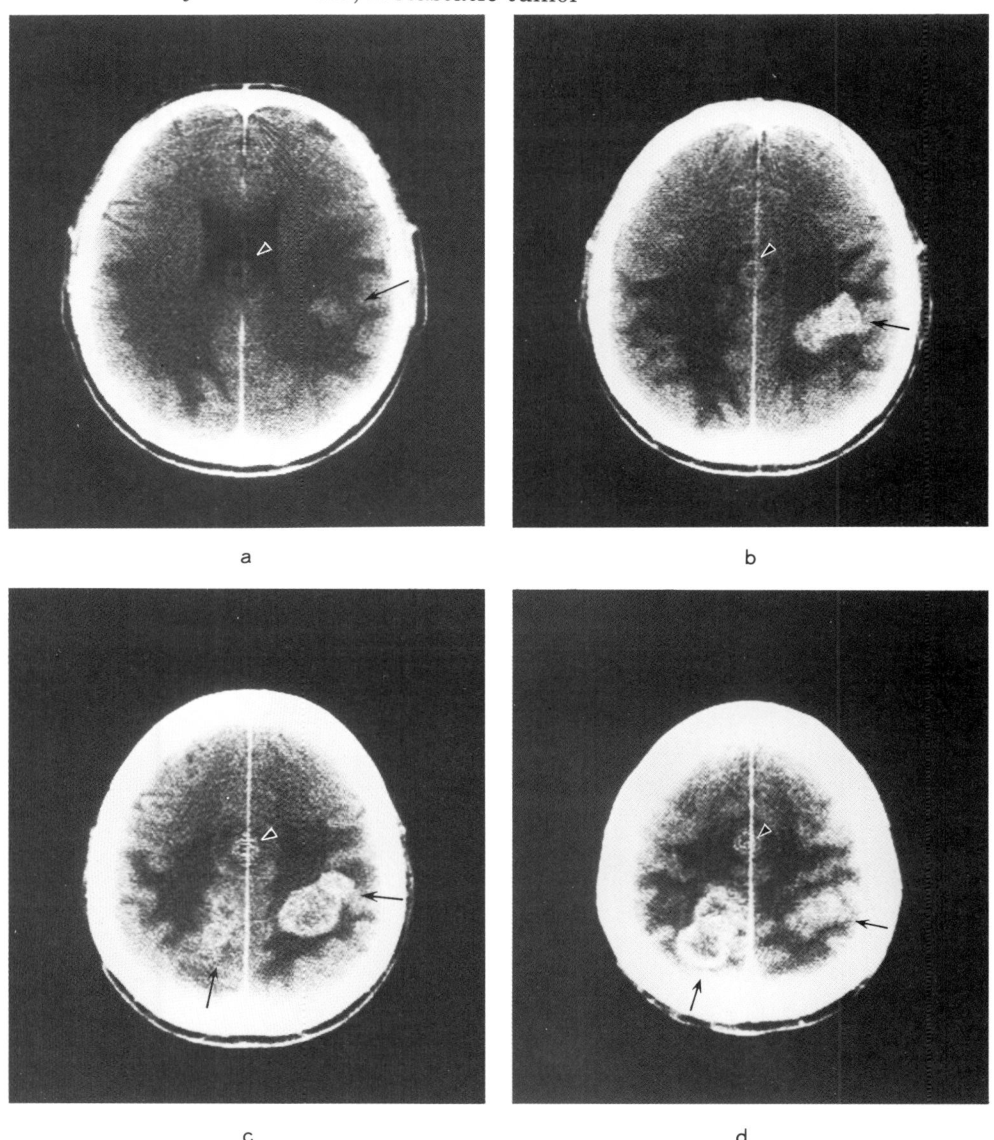

Fig. 92

This patient's history was unremarkable. His primary complaint was reduced muscle strength in the extremities, which began a month before examination. He also felt "heavy-headed". On first examination, the patient was lucid but showed bilateral papilledema and tetraparesis in the extremities. CT scans revealed many tumors (←) in both cerebral hemispheres which are of high absorption due to uptake of intravenously administered iodine solution. Wide low-absorption areas caused by brain edema surrounded the tumorous regions. The tumor originated in the kidney and was demonstrated on physical examination. A ring shadow indicated by the arrow head (◁) is an artifact.

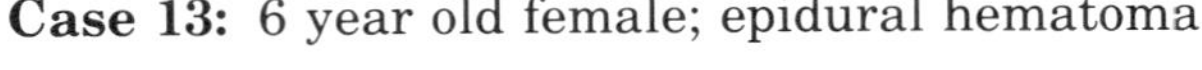

Case 13: 6 year old female; epidural hematoma

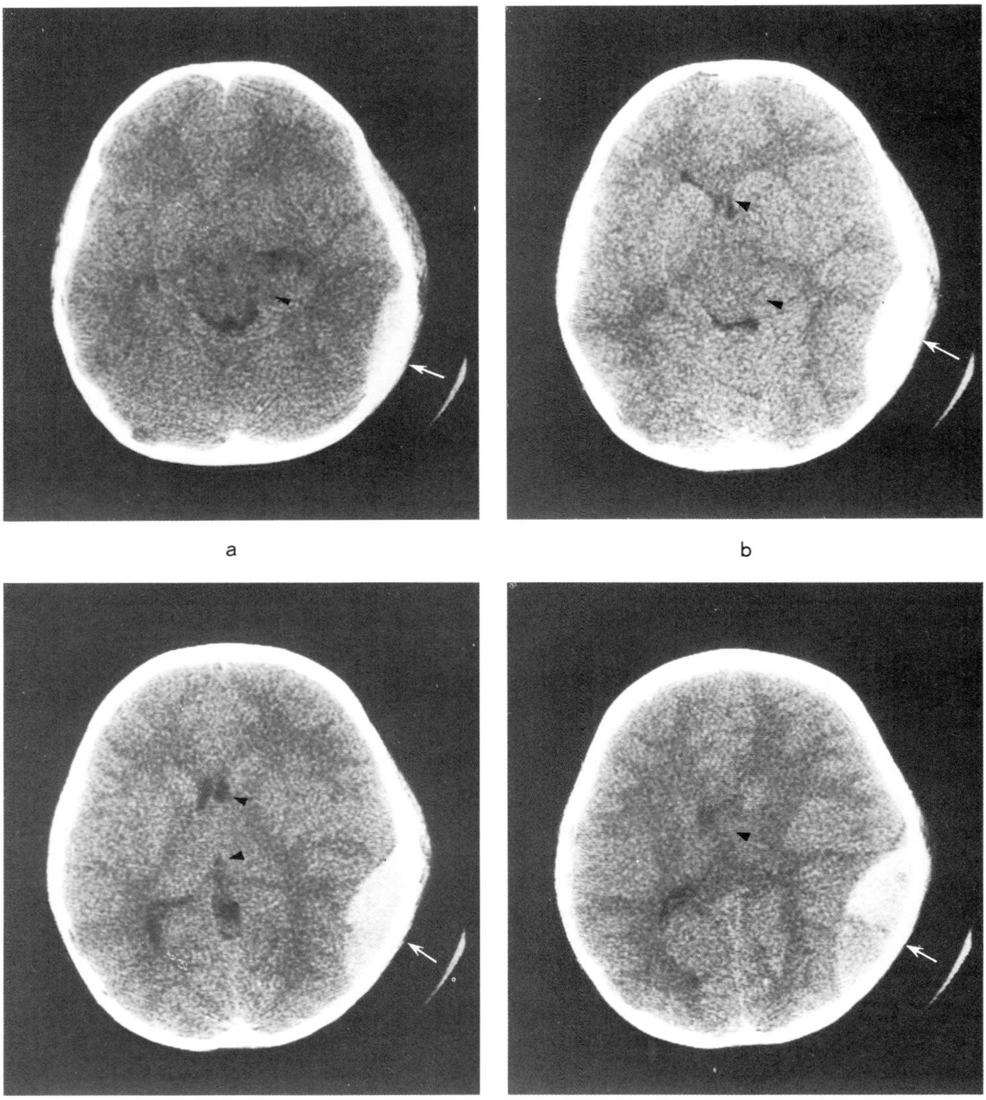

a

b

c

d

Fig. 93

While playing, this patient was hit in the right temporal region by a car. The patient remained conscious after the accident, but she began vomiting repeatedly after two days. When transferred for the present examination, three days after the accident, she was lethargic. The only neurological abnormalities observed were increased tendon reflexes on the left side.

CT scans revealed a lens-shaped high absorption area in the right temporal-parietal region (←). The ventricles were displaced and deformed, with a compensatory dislocation to the contralateral side (◀).

Case 14: 29 year old male, meningioma

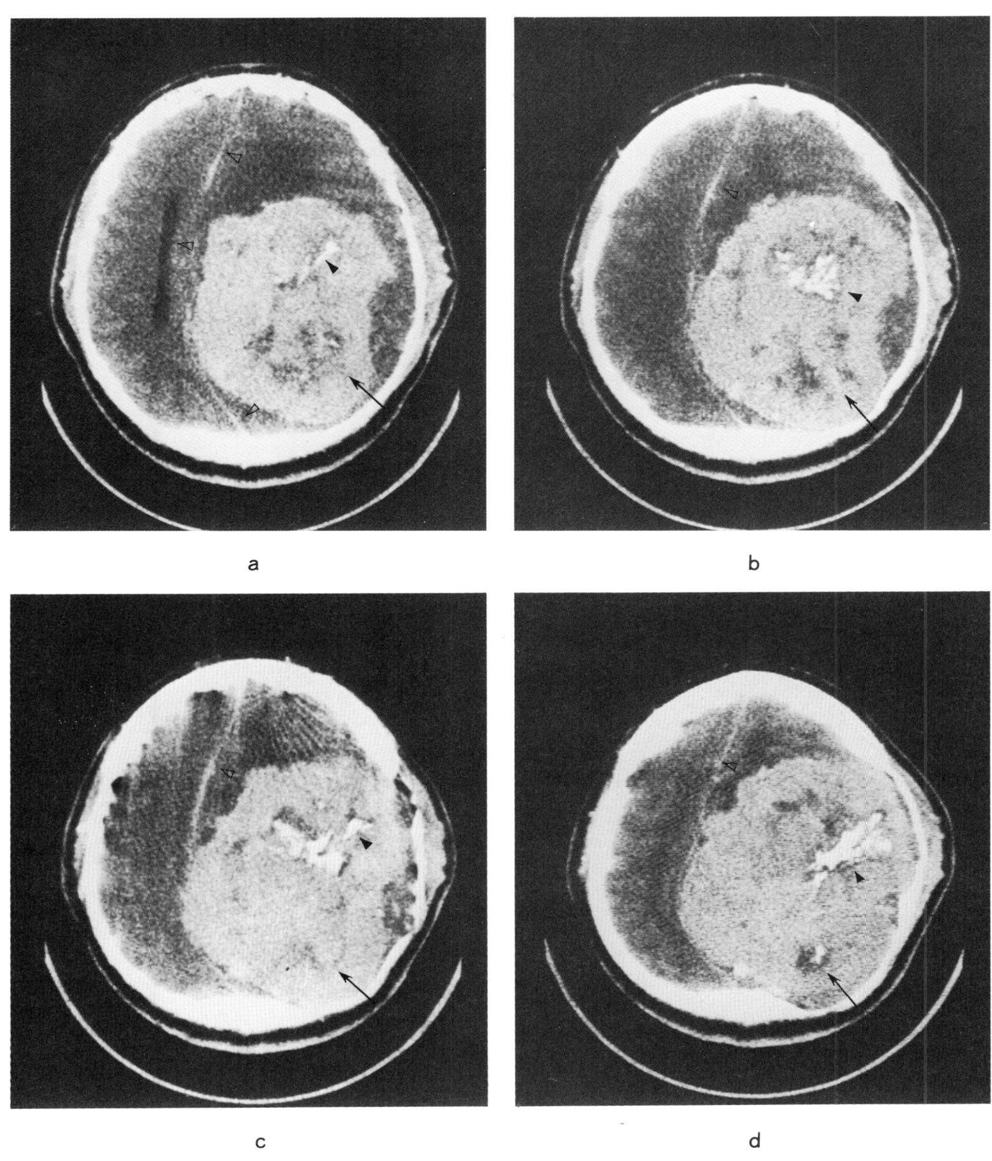

a b c d

Fig. 94

Five years before the present examination and just after an epileptic fit, this patient had been informed of an intracranial tumor. However, he was fearful of surgical removal and insisted upon conservative treatment. Bilateral papilledema was observed. After hospitalization, he could not stand up because of stupor and left-sided hemiplegia.

CT scans after intravenous contrast injection revealed a large tumor of high absorption occupying virtually all of the right parietal region (←). In addition, calcification was detected within the tumor (◀). Note that the ventricles and falx were severely pushed to the contralateral side (◁).

6. CRANIAL NERVES AND THEIR FUNCTIONS

There are 12 pairs of cranial nerves, each with a name and a number. The numbers represent the rostral-caudal order in which each nerve penetrates the dura mater (Fig. 96). Table 8 will aid in the memorization of these names and numbers. Each nerve is subsequently described in detail. This information is difficult for most students to master but it is essential to look through Table 9, Figure 95 and summary of the cranial nerves for understanding the basic features of the cranial nerves.

Table 8.

On Old Olympus' Towering Top, A Finn And German Viewed Some Hops.

Table 9. CRANIAL NERVES AND THEIR FUNCTIONS

I. Olfactory nerve: smell
II. Optic nerve: sight
III. Oculomotor nerve: eye movement, pupil changes
IV. Trochlear nerve: eye movement
V. Trigeminal nerve: chewing, sensations about the head
VI. Abducens nerve: eye movement
VII. Facial nerve: facial muscle movement, lacrimal gland, taste, salivary gland
VIII. Vestibulocochlear nerve: hearing, posture
IX. Glossopharyngeal nerve: taste, salivary gland, swallowing, carotid sinus and body
X. Vagus nerve: parasympathetic nerve (visceral muscle movement), swallowing, articulation in speaking
XI. (Spinal) Accessory nerve: head and shoulder movement
XII. Hypoglossal nerve: tongue movement

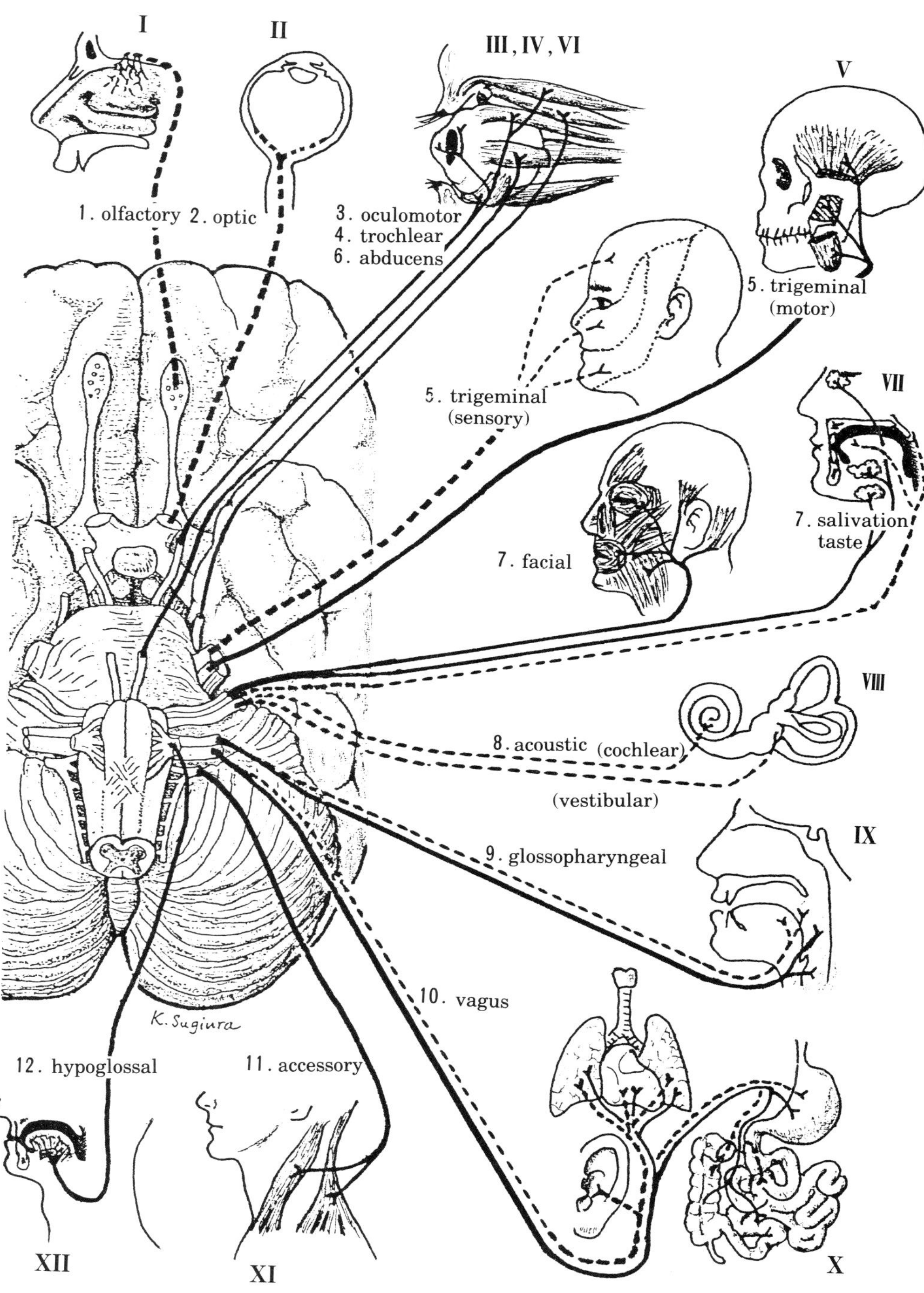

Fig. 95 Cranial nerves and their functions (modified from Netter).

SUMMARY OF THE CRANIAL NERVES

1. All the cranial nerves exit from foramina in the skull. However, their origins are not always in the brain. Most of the accessory nerve fibers originate in the spinal cord.
2. Organs supplied by the cranial nerves are in the head and neck, except for those supplied by the vagus (X).
3. Cranial nerves penetrate foramina in the skull on the way to their targets. These foramina are all located in the cranial base (Fig. 96). As a result, damage to the cranial nerves is common after injury to this area (e.g., basal skull fracture).

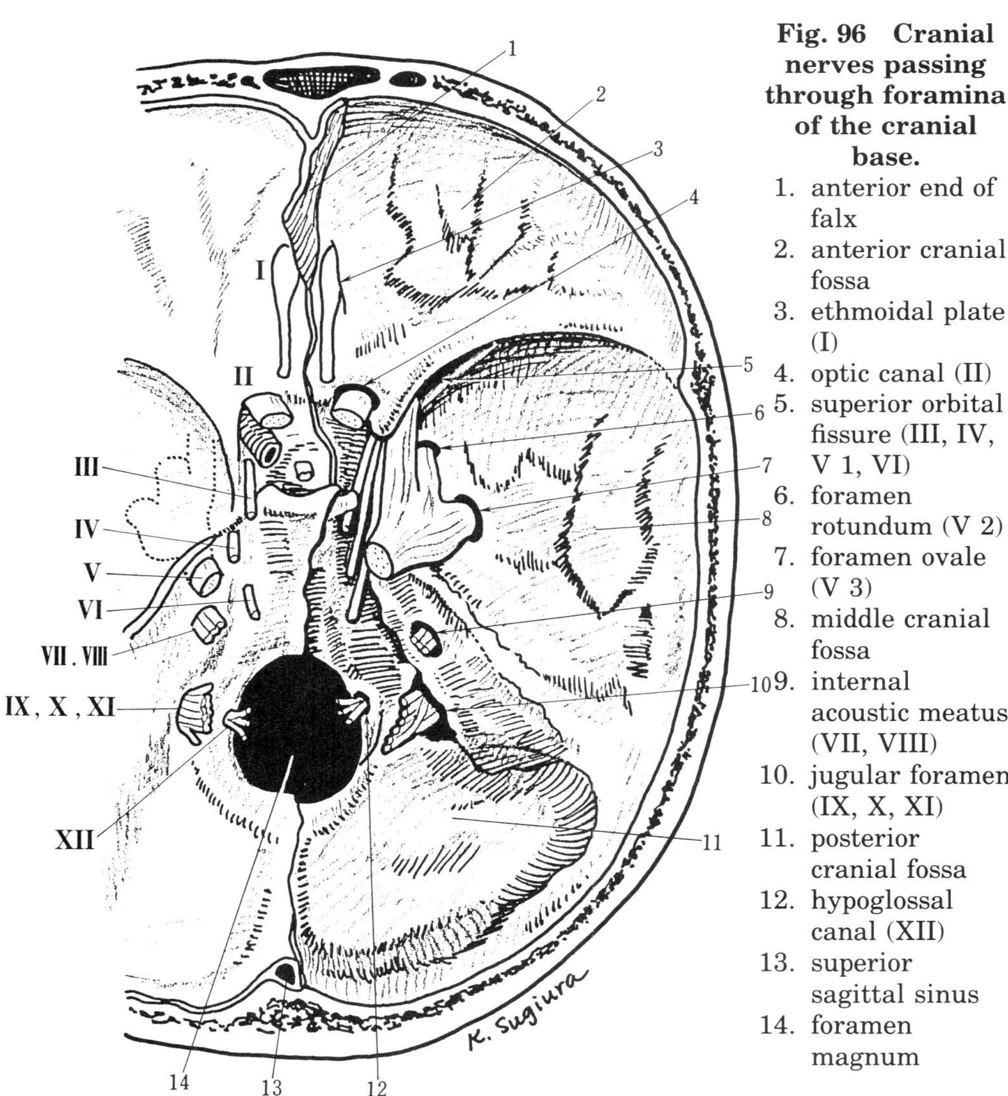

Fig. 96 Cranial nerves passing through foramina of the cranial base.

1. anterior end of falx
2. anterior cranial fossa
3. ethmoidal plate (I)
4. optic canal (II)
5. superior orbital fissure (III, IV, V 1, VI)
6. foramen rotundum (V 2)
7. foramen ovale (V 3)
8. middle cranial fossa
9. internal acoustic meatus (VII, VIII)
10. jugular foramen (IX, X, XI)
11. posterior cranial fossa
12. hypoglossal canal (XII)
13. superior sagittal sinus
14. foramen magnum

4. Before penetrating the cranial foramina, the cranial nerves must pass through the dura mater. These two exits are sometimes apart of each other, particularly in the case of the IIIrd, IVth, Vth and VIth nerves (Fig. 96). They all course a short distance in the cavernous sinus before leaving the skull.
5. Cranial nerves originate on the ventral side of the brain, except for the trochlear nerve (IV) (Fig. 97) which begins on the dorsal side of the midbrain and then courses toward the ventral side (Fig. 69).

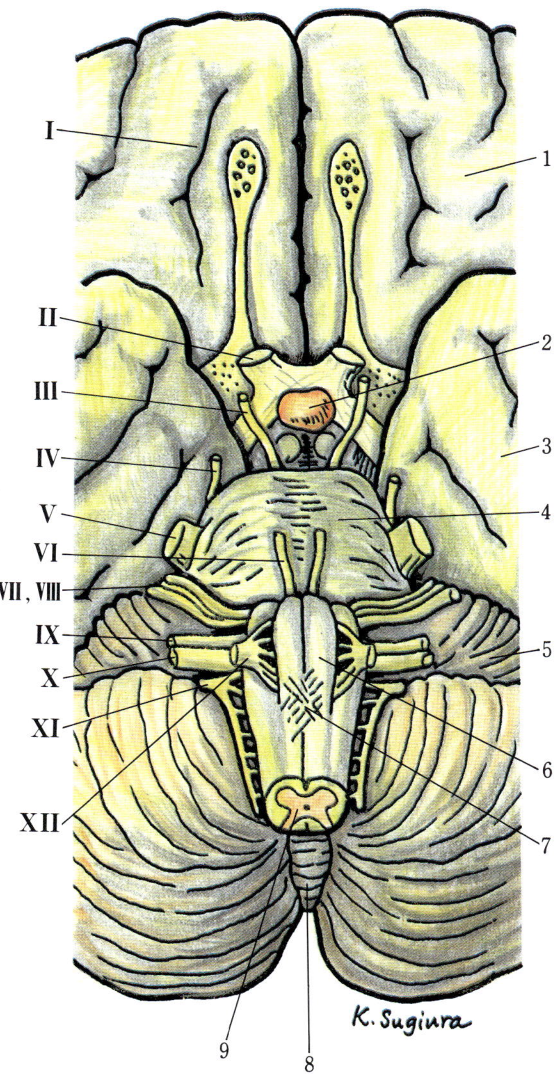

Fig. 97 Cranial nerves at the base of the brain.

1. frontal lobe
2. hypophysis
3. temporal lobe
4. pons
5. cerebellar hemisphere
6. pyramid (medulla)
7. pyramidal decussation
8. vermis of cerebellum
9. spinal cord

6. Nuclei of the cranial nerves are located in the brain stem (midbrain, pons, medulla) except for I, II and XI, as shown in Fig. 98. As mentioned above, paralysis of the cranial nerves often follows lesions of the brain stem.
7. In addition to sensory and motor fibers, the cranial nerves contain autonomic fibers.
8. Autonomic fibers in cranial nerves belong to the parasympathetic nervous system, with most in the vagus nerve (X), and the rest in III, VII and IX.
9. Pure sensory nerves are in three pairs (I, II, VIII), and pure motor nerves are in four pairs (IV, VI, XI, XII). Five of the remaining pairs (III, V, VII, IX, X) are mixed with sensory, motor or parasympathetic fibers.

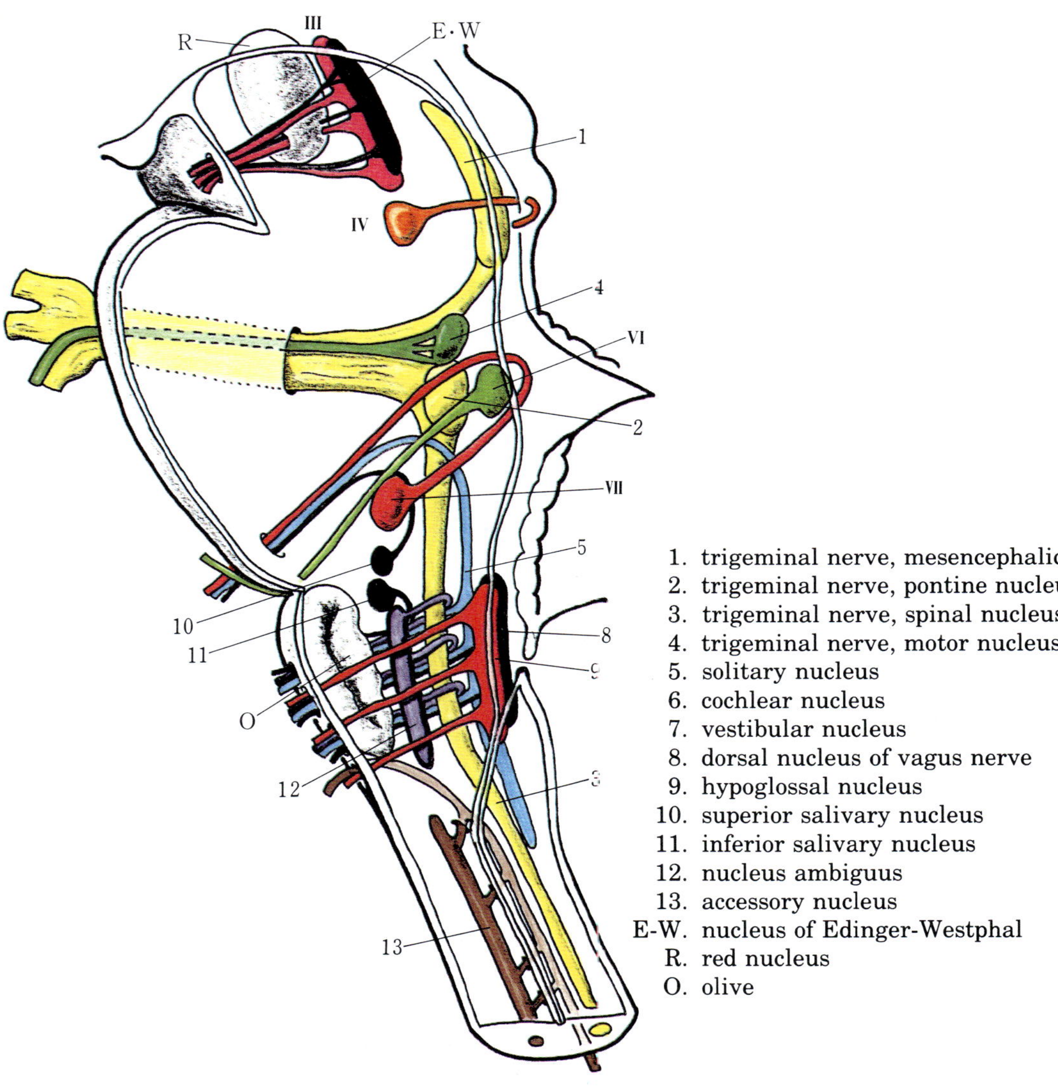

Fig. 98 Nuclei of the cranial nerves. A. lateral view

10. Nuclei of cranial motor nerves are under the control of the frontal lobe. Fibers from this lobe descend in the pyramidal tract to the internal capsule, pass through the cerebral peduncles and into the brain stem where they cross the midline just before reaching the nuclei. This contralateral distribution is typically seen only in lower facial muscles (i.e., innervated by VII). Other cranial nuclei are controlled, in addition, by non-crossing frontal-lobe projections. As a result, symptoms of a unilateral supranculear disorder are clear only for the lower face region (VII).
11. Table 10 provides a summary about the cranial nerves. It should be studied last, to reinforce the points made above.

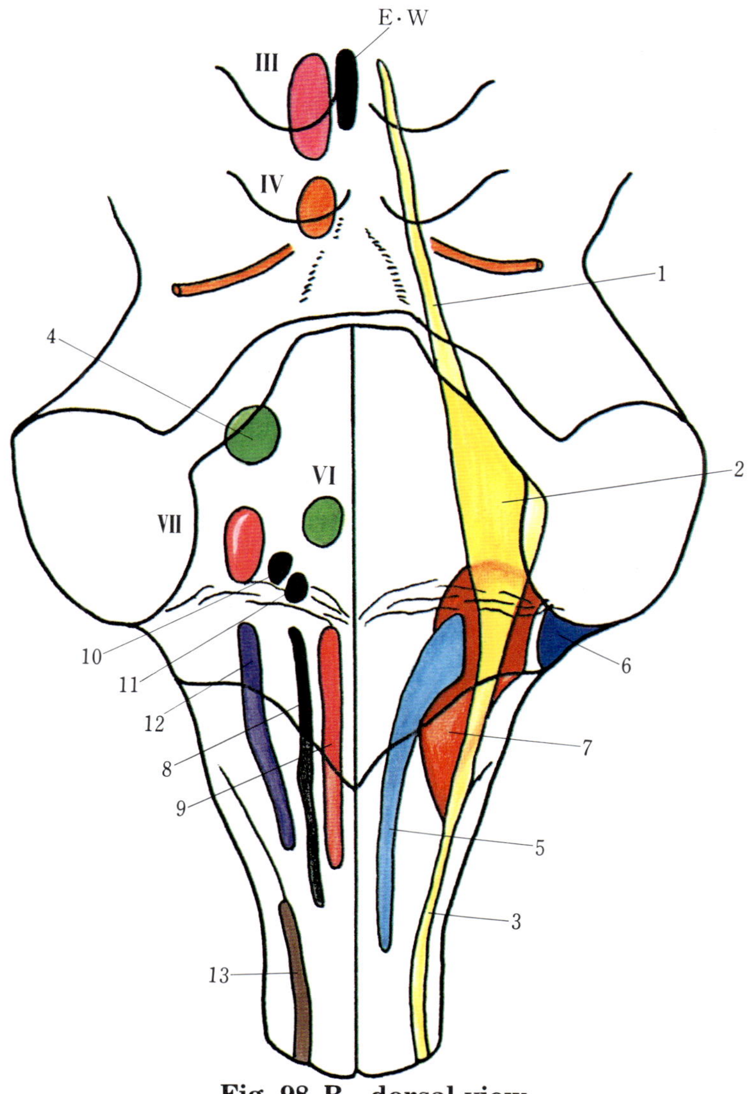

Fig. 98 B dorsal view
Motor and sensory nuclei are shown on the left and right sides, respectively.

Table 10 Cranial nerves and their functions

nerve	effective organ	foramen of the skull	origin at the brain	nucleus	intermediate pathway (nucleus)	center	function
I Olfactory	sensory: olfactory epithelium	→ ethmoidal plate	→ olfactory triangle	(—)		temporal lobe	sense of smell
II Optic	sensory: retina	→ optic canal	→ diencephalon	→ { pretectal area	→ E·W nucleus → Oculomotor nerve		light reflex
				lateral geniculate body }	→ posterior limb of internal capsule → optic radiation	→ occiptal lobe	vision
III Oculomotor	motor: sup. rectus, inf. rectus, med. rectus, inf. obliquus and levator palpebrae muscle	← superior orbital fissure	← ventral side of midbrain	← oculomotor nucleus (midbrain)	← (MLF) ← (center for fixation)	← frontal and occipital lobe	motion of eye
	autonomic: sphincter	←	←	← E·W nucleus (midbrain)	←	← hypothalamus	pupil constriction
IV Trochlear	motor: sup. obliquus muscle	← superior orbital fissure	← dorsal side of midbrain	← trochlear nucleus (midbrain)	← (MLF) ← (center for fixation)	← frontal and occipital lobe	motion of eye
V Trigeminal	sensory: face, mucous membrane of nasal and oral cavity (tongue), cornea	→ { sup. orbital fissure (1) foramen rotundum (2) foramen ovale (3) }	→ pons	→ pontine nucleus of trigeminal nerve (pons)	→ thalamus	→ parietal lobe	facial tactile
				→ spinal nucleus (pons ~ spinal cord)			facial pain—temperature
				→ mesencephalic nucleus (midbrain)			facial proprioception
	motor: masticatory muscles	← foramen ovale	←	← motor nucleus of trigeminal nerve (pons)	← internal capsule	← frontal lobe	mastication
VI Abducens	motor: lateral rectus muscle	← superior orbital fissure	← between pons and medulla	← abducens nucleus (pons)	← (MLF) ← (center for fixation)	← frontal and occipital lobe	motion of eye
VII Facial	motor: facial muscles	← stylomastoid foramen ↑	←	← facial nucleus (pons)	← internal capsule	← frontal lobe	facial movement
	sensory: anterior ⅔ taste buds, corda tympani	→ internal acoustic meatus	→ between pons and medulla	→ solitary nucleus (pons < medulla)	→ thalamus	→ parietal lobe	taste, anterior ⅔ of tongue
	autonomic: submandibular, sublingual and lacrimal gland, corda tympani	←	←	← superior salivary nucleus (pons)	←	← hypothalamus	secretion of saliva and tears
VIII Vestibulo-cochlear	sensory: semicircular canal, utricle, saccule, Corti's organ	→ internal acoustic meatus	→ between pons and medulla	→ { vestibular nucleus (pons)	→ connection with cerebellum/motor system	→ (temporal lobe)	equilibrium acceleration
				cochlear nucleus (pons) }	→ lateral lemniscus → inferior colliculi → medial geniculate body	→ temporal lobe	hearing
IX Glossopharyngeal	sensory: pharynx and larynx mucous membrane, Eustachian tube, internal ear, carotid body, posterior ⅓ of tongue taste buds	→ jugular foramen	→ medulla oblongata	→ { spinal nucleus of trigeminal nerve solitary nucleus (pons < medulla) }	→ thalamus → formation of autonomic reflex arc	→ parietal lobe	sense in pharynx and larynx.
	motor: muscles in larynx and pharynx	←	←	← nucleus ambiguus (medulla)	← internal capsule	← frontal lobe	movement of pharynx and larynx
	autonomic: parotid gland	←	←	← inferior salivary nucleus (medulla)	←	← hypothalamus	secretion of saliva
X Vagus	autonomic: organs in thorax and abdomen	←	←	← dorsal nucleus of vagus (medulla)	←	← hypothalamus	viscera
	motor: muscles in pharynx and larynx	← jugular foramen	← medulla oblongata	← nucleus ambiguus (medulla)	← internal capsule	← frontal lobe	movement of pharynx and larynx
	sensory: auricle, external acoustic meatus, viscera	→	→	→ spinal nucleus of trigeminal nerve solitary nucleus (medulla)	→ thalamus → formation of autonomic reflex arc	→ parietal lobe	pain—temperature of ear
XI Accessory	motor: sternocleidomastoid muscle, trapezoid muscle	← jugular foramen	← medulla, spinal cord	← accessory nucleus (medulla < cervical cord)	← internal capsule	← frontal lobe	neck movement
XII Hypoglossal	motor: muscles in tongue	← hypoglossal canal	← medulla	← hypoglossal nucleus (medulla)	← internal capsule	← frontal lobe	tongue movement

OLFACTORY NERVE (I)

This is a pure sensory nerve, serving the sense of smell. The stimuli received by the mucous membranes of the nasal cavity are registered by olfactory filaments (99–1) which enter the cranium through the cribriform plate in the anterior cranial base. Impulses are conducted to the olfactory tract (99–3), and finally reach the amygdala (99–4) and the hippocampus (99–5) in the temporal lobe.

The olfactory filaments are occasionally broken and anosmia may occur after head trauma (especially a basal skull fracture) or after an operation involving the anterior cranial base. Anosmia is not only an inconvenience in daily life, but it also causes a lack of appetite and susceptibility to accidental gas intoxication, because the subject is not aware of the harmful agent.

Damage to the olfactory filaments may also cause cerebrospinal fluid (CSF) rhinorrhea. This involves not only CSF leaking through the cribriform plate, but also the occasional meningitis.

Bone of the anterior cranial base, on which the olfactory tract lies, is concave and called the olfactory groove. It is a common site for the growth of a meningioma. Stimulation of the temporal lobe can cause an uncinate fit, as described previously.

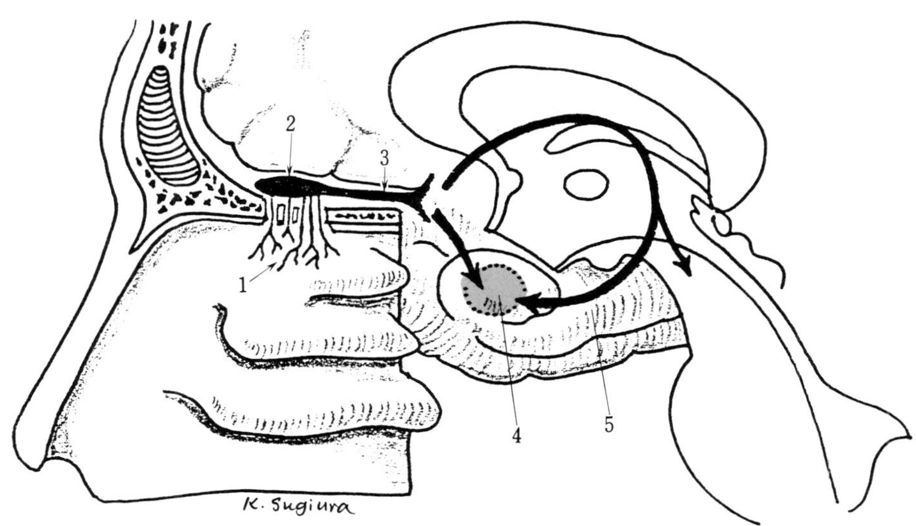

Fig. 99 The olfactory nerve.
1. olfactory striae
2. olfactory bulb
3. olfactory tract
4. amygdala
5. hippocampus

OPTIC NERVE (II)

The assessment of visual acuity, field of vision and the retina are the most important parts of the neurological examination.

The optic nerve is also a pure sensory (photoreception) cranial nerve. Sensory input from the retina enters the cranium antero-laterally to the sella turcica via the optic nerve (100–2) and optic canal (100–3). The optic chiasm (100–4) is found anterior and superior to the sella. It is a semi-decussation, with axons supplying the medial half of the retina crossing to the other side and axons supplying the lateral half remaining ipsilateral (Figs. 101, 102). Therefore, sensory information about the right field of vision enters the left optic tract (100–5) and that of the left field enters the right tract. It is essential to remember that the up-down and left-right relations between the field of vision and the projection patterns of optic-nerve axons are completely reversed posterior to the chiasm.

Optic-tract axons that participate in vision project to the lateral geniculate body (100–6, 101–1, 102), a part of the thalamus. The next-order axons form the optic radiations (100–7) which project to the occipital lobe (100–8).

Other optic-tract axons participate in the light reflex. They do not project to the lateral geniculate body, but rather, to the Edinger-Westphal nucleus (101–4) in the pretectal area. The next-order axons from this nucleus project to the oculomotor nucleus (101–6) bilaterally, after which there is a motor output to the sphincter pupillae muscle by way of the oculomotor nerve (101–7). The light reflex, which serves to regulate pupil diameter, has a bilateral output (i.e., increased light to one eye reduces pupil diameter in both eyes). This is important when using the light reflex to determine the location of a lesion (Fig. 101).

Abnormalities of the visual field provide important information about the location of brain lesions. Damage to an optic nerve can cause loss of sight in one eye (102–A). Bitemporal hemianopia (102–B) and binasal hemianopia only occur when there is

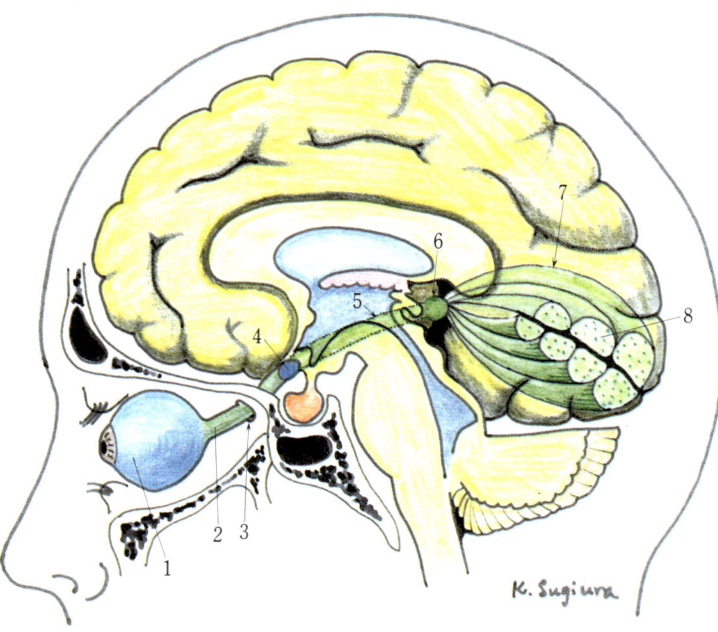

Fig. 100 Pathways of the optic nerve.
1. eye
2. optic nerve
3. optic canal
4. optic chiasm
5. optic tract
6. lateral geniculate body
7. optic radiation
8. visual cortex of the occipital lobe

damage to the optic chiasm. Both homonymous hemianopia (102–D) and quadrantanopia (102–E, F) indicate that the lesion is at or posterior to the optic tract. A lesion close to the visual cortex typically causes a deficit in which the central visual field remains unaffected (macular sparing, 102–G).

Papilledema or choked disc, as a symptom of increased intracranial pressure, will be described later.

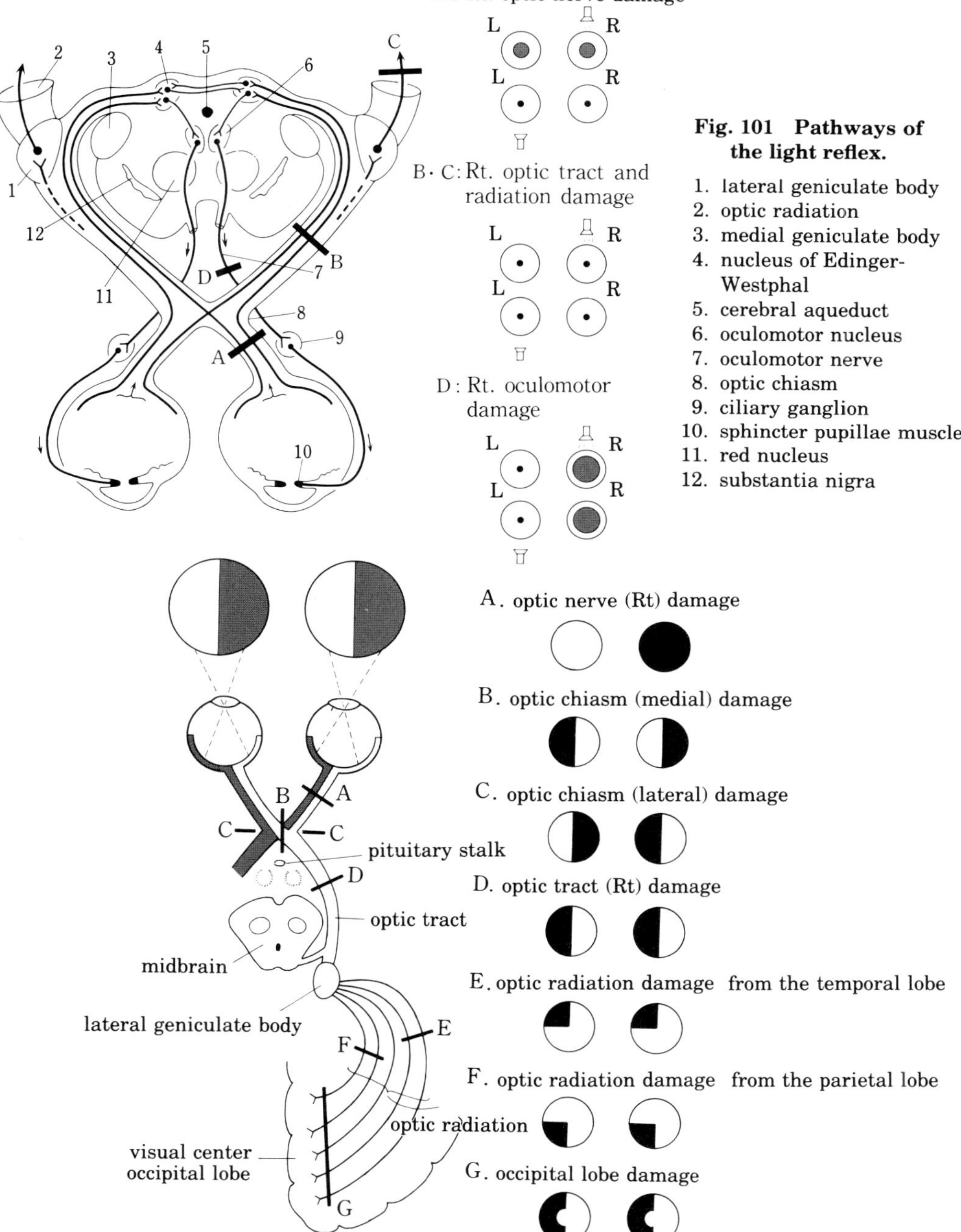

Fig. 101 Pathways of the light reflex.

1. lateral geniculate body
2. optic radiation
3. medial geniculate body
4. nucleus of Edinger-Westphal
5. cerebral aqueduct
6. oculomotor nucleus
7. oculomotor nerve
8. optic chiasm
9. ciliary ganglion
10. sphincter pupillae muscle
11. red nucleus
12. substantia nigra

Fig. 102 Visual field deficits resulting from selected lesions.

OCULOMOTOR (III), TROCHLEAR (IV) AND ABDUCENS (VI) NERVES

Eye movements are carried out by combinations of delicate contractions and relaxations of the extrinsic muscles of the eyeballs, which are supplied by the oculomotor, trochlear and abducens nerves. These are almost pure motor nerves except for the oculomotor nerve, which includes autonomic fibers to the pupil.

The extrinsic muscles include the superior and inferior oblique, and the superior, inferior, medial and lateral rectus muscles. The superior oblique and lateral rectus are supplied by the trochlear and abducens nerves, respectively. All others are innervated by the oculomotor nerve which also supplies the levator palpebrae and pupillary constrictor muscles.

The oculomotor nerve (104–III) originates in the oculomotor nucleus (101–6) of the midbrain. It emerges between the cerebral peduncles, proceeds under the posterior cerebral artery (104–5) and penetrates the dura mater lateral to the clivus. Finally, it enters the cavernous sinus (103, 104–2). The trochlear nerve (104–IV) originates in the trochlear nucleus (also of the midbrain). It emerges from the posterior midbrain at the level of the inferior colliculus, then crosses to the contralateral side, where it circumvents the cerebral peduncle, and penetrates the dura mater lateral and posterior to the oculomotor nerve. Finally, it too enters the cavernous

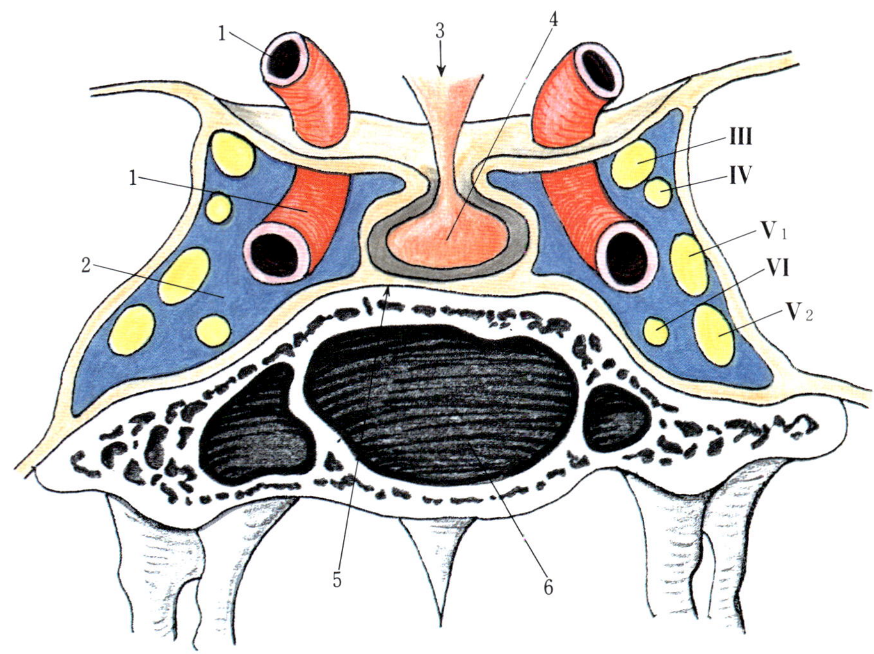

Fig. 103 The cavernous sinus.

1. internal carotid artery
2. cavernous sinus
3. infundibulum
4. hypophysis
5. base of the sella turcica
6. sphenoidal sinus

III. oculomotor nerve
IV. trochlear nerve
V1. trigeminal nerve, first branch
V2. trigeminal nerve, second branch
VI. abducens nerve

sinus. The abducens nucleus is located in the pons (104–3), caudal of course to the oculomotor and trochlear nuclei. The abducens nerve (104–VI) runs within the pons in an antero-inferior direction, to leave the brain stem close to the midline between the pons and medulla. Next, it proceeds for a relatively long distance within the subarachnoid space between the pons and the clivus, before penetrating the dura mater medial and posterior to the trochlear nerve, to enter the cavernous sinus. Abducens nerve paralysis frequently accompanies increased intracranial pressure, probably due to its relatively long path in the subarachnoid space.

Thus, the cavernous sinus (Figs. 103, 104—2) accommodates the oculomotor, trochlear and abducens nerves. They enter the orbital cavity through the superior orbital fissure (104—1) from which they project towards their target muscles. Also traversing the cavernous sinus are the first and the second branches of the trigeminal nerve and the internal carotid artery (Figs. 103, 104). As a result, a lesion in the cavernous sinus or in the superior orbital fissure, such as a carotid-cavernous fistula (CCF), can simultaneously compress nerves III, IV, V and VI (the cavernous sinus syndrome).

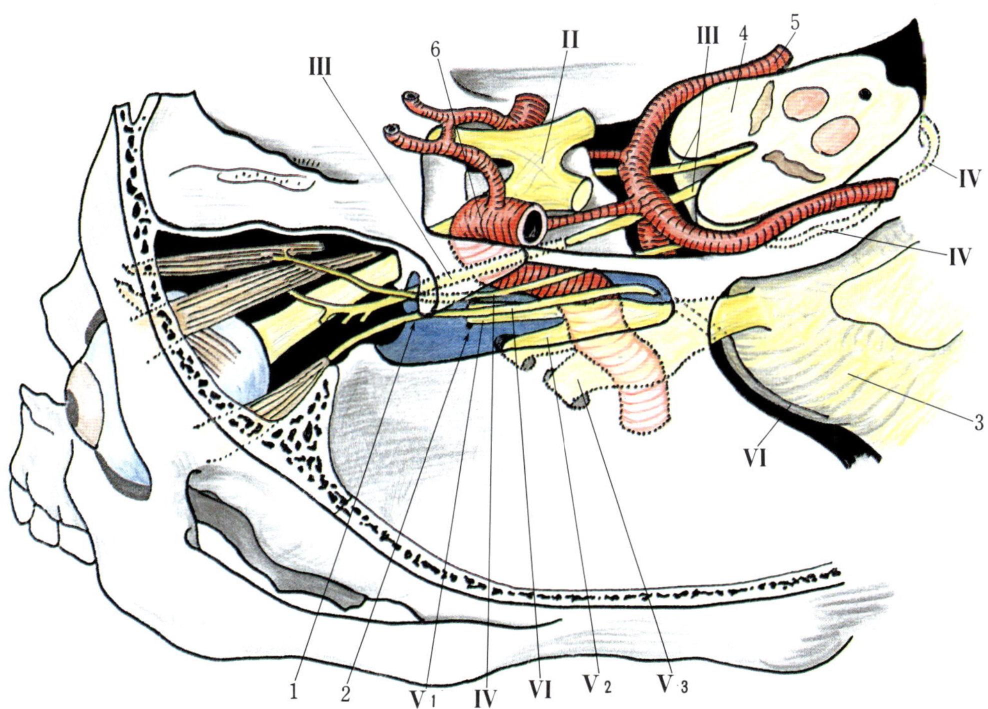

Fig. 104 Anatomy of cranial base (from Patten).

1. superior orbital fissure
2. cavernous sinus
3. pons
4. midbrain (cerebral peduncle)
5. posterior cerebral artery
6. internal carotid artery

II. optic chiasm
III. oculomotor nerve
IV. trochlear nerve
V1. trigeminal nerve, first branch
V2. trigeminal nerve, second branch
V3. trigeminal nerve, third branch
VI. abducens nerve

Normally, the oculomotor, trochlear and abducens nerves do not function independently. Consider directing the eyes to the right. For this task, the active muscles are mainly the lateral rectus (abducens) of the right eye and the medial rectus (oculomotor) of the left eye. However, the right medial rectus (oculomotor) and the left lateral rectus (abducens) must be relaxed for both eyes to turn rightwards (Fig. 105). Thus, a complex control system is needed to move both eyes in the same direction (i.e., to gaze).

The cerebral centers for eye movements are located in the eye-movement areas of the frontal and the occipital lobes. However, these are not sufficient to produce accurate movements. Other requisite centers are called the subcortical centers for fixation. These include centers for perpendicular fixation and convergence (106–2) in the pretectal region of the midbrain and the center for horizontal fixation near the abducens nucleus in the pons (accessory abducens nucleus, 106–7). These subcortical centers and the eye-movement nuclei (III, IV, VI) are inter-connected by fibers of the medial longitudinal fasciculus (MLF) (106–5), located in the brain stem.

A disorder in the pretectal region caused, for example, by a tumor of the pineal body (106–1) brings on a paralysis of perpendicular fixation and convergence, a symptom known as Parinaud's syndrome (107–B).

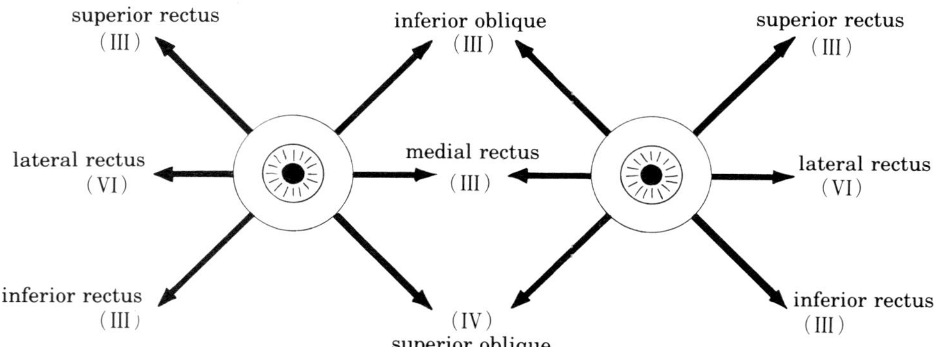

Fig. 105 Function and innervation of the extra-ocular muscles, nerve supply in parentheses.

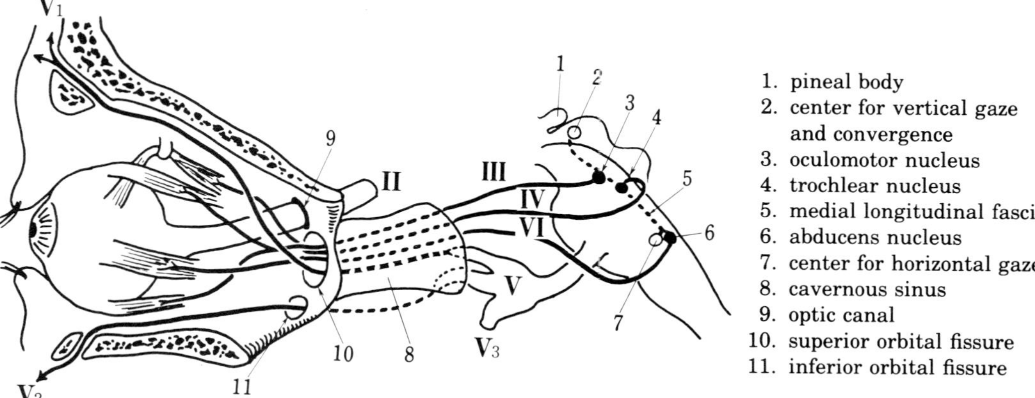

Fig. 106 Pathways of nerves controlling movement of the eye: Branches of the trigeminal nerve and the cavernous sinus are also shown.

A lesion in the accessory abducens nucleus of the pons causes deviation of the eyes to the contralateral side of the lesion (conjugate deviation, 107–C). The patient cannot gaze toward the side of the lesion, a deficit called Foville's syndrome.

Fig. 105 shows the relationship between extrinsic muscles and the direction of eye movements. For example, in the case of a right abducens nerve palsy (107–D), the right eye takes on a position of adduction (strabism). This is accompanied by double vision (diplopia), observed typically during gazing toward the right side. Strabism and diplopia caused by trochlear nerve palsy (involving paralysis of the superior oblique muscle) are not so obvious, and might be compensated for by other muscles over time.

Oculomotor nerve palsy (107–E) on the right side causes deviation of the right eye to the right due to unopposed tone contraction of the normal lateral rectus muscle, and double vision, which is most severe during gazing toward the left. Since the oculomotor nerve supplies the levator palpebrae superioris and the sphincter pupillae muscles, ptosis and pupillary dilatation may be observed on the right side. The asymmetry of both pupils observed in this case is generally called anisocoria. Thus, oculomotor nerve palsy participates in Weber's syndrome (a midbrain disorder), of concern not only in internal medicine, but also in neurosurgery as a potentially important symptom of an internal carotid—posterior communicating artery aneurysm.

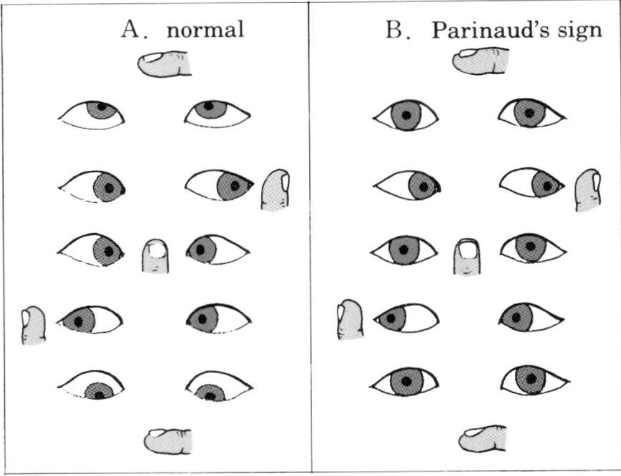

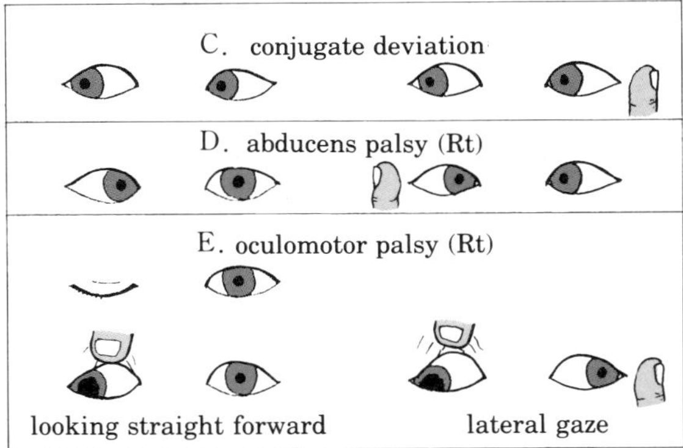

Fig. 107 Disorders of eye movements.

TRIGEMINAL NERVE (V)

The trigeminal nerve has sensory fibers from the face and motor fibers to muscles of mastication. The name, trigeminal, comes from its three projections from the trigeminal ganglion (also called the semilunar or Gasserian ganglion, 108–7). The first branch (also called the ophthalmic nerve, 108–V1) conducts sensory input from the frontal skin and the cornea to the trigeminal ganglion, by way of the orbital cavity, superior orbital fissure, and cavernous sinus. The second branch (maxillary nerve, 108–V2) contains sensory fibers from maxillary skin and from nasal mucous membranes. These pass through the orbital cavity, inferior orbital fissure, foramen rotundum, and cavernous sinus. The third branch (mandibular nerve, 108–V3) conveys sensory input from the lower jaw and tongue to the trigeminal ganglion by way of the foramen ovale. Central to the ganglion is a single thick bundle of fibers which enters the brain stem on the lateral side of the pons to terminate in the trigeminal nuclei, as described below.

The trigeminal nucleus in the brain stem is divided into four parts: the principal sensory nucleus (pontine nucleus, 108–5) receiving tactile input, the mesencephalic nucleus (108–4) receiving proprioceptive input, the spinal nucleus (108–6) receiving pain-temperature input and the trigeminal motor nucleus (108–5) which sends fibers to the muscles of mastication (108–8). Projections from the former three nuclei cross to the contralateral side, to reach the ventro-posteromedial nucleus of the thalamus. Axons to the muscles of mastication emerge from the trigeminal motor nucleus and exit the cranium via the foramen ovale, travelling with the third (mandibular) branch of the trigeminal nerve.

A well-known disorder of the trigeminal nerve is trigeminal neuralgia, or tic doloureux. It brings on short episodes of severe pain limited to a small part of the face supplied by one or two trigeminal branches. The nature and intensity of the pain is described as being similar to that of dental treatment without anesthesia. Its cause is unknown, but one possibility in certain cases is that mechanical activation of the nerve within the posterior cranial fossa may occur due to convoluted blood vessels. Essential trigeminal neuralgia (i.e., tic doloureux) should be distinguished from other pathological cases involving this nerve, for example, where shingles or tumors are involved.

The first of the three trigeminal branches is the most important clinically, because it is involved with corneal sensation. When this branch is damaged, the corneal reflex is abolished and pain will not be perceived. A patient with this problem does not try to remove foreign material from the eye. Consequently, the cornea becomes inflamed and is predisposed to ulcerative perforation and loss of vision.

Sometimes, the second or third branch of the trigeminal nerve may be cut for therapeutic purposes. However, effort should be made to maintain the first branch as long as possible.

(SPINAL NUCLEUS OF THE TRIGEMINAL NERVE AND HEADACHE)

The spinal nucleus (108–6) extends inferiorly from the pontine level to the third or fourth segments of the cervical cord. This is a relay nucleus where pain-temperature input is integrated from the face, the dura mater and large blood vessels of the brain, eyeball (cornea), ear, paranasal cavities, oral cavity and tongue. In addition, this nucleus may receive input from the pharynx and larynx (via the glossopharyngeal and vagus nerves) and from the dorsal roots of the second and third cervical nerves (concerning sensation in the occipital and nuchal areas). Thus, virtually all headaches attributable to intracranial disturbances involve sensory input to the brain by way of the spinal nucleus of the trigeminal nerve. Such trigeminally mediated headaches often accompany pain in the eye, ear, nose (paranasal cavity), mouth (toothache), temporo-mandibular joint and nuchal area.

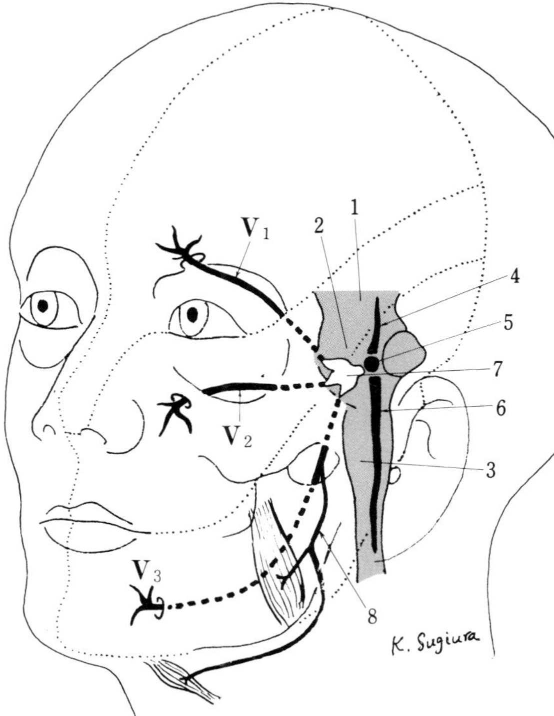

Fig. 108 Distribution of the trigeminal nerve.
Figs. 104 and 106 show the relation between the cavernous sinus and the three branches of the trigeminal nerve.

1. midbrain
2. pons
3. medulla oblongata
4. mesencephalic nucleus (V)
5. pontine and motor nuclei (V)
6. spinal nucleus (V)
7. semilunar ganglion
8. fibers to muscles of mastication

V1. first branch (ophthalmic nerve)
V2. second branch (maxillary nerve)
V3. third branch (mandibular nerve)

(THE CORNEAL REFLEX (109))

This reflex brings about eyelid closure when the cornea is touched gently. The afferent pathway is the first branch of the trigeminal nerve. The efferent pathway is the facial nerve. Damage to either nerve abolishes or reduces this reflex.

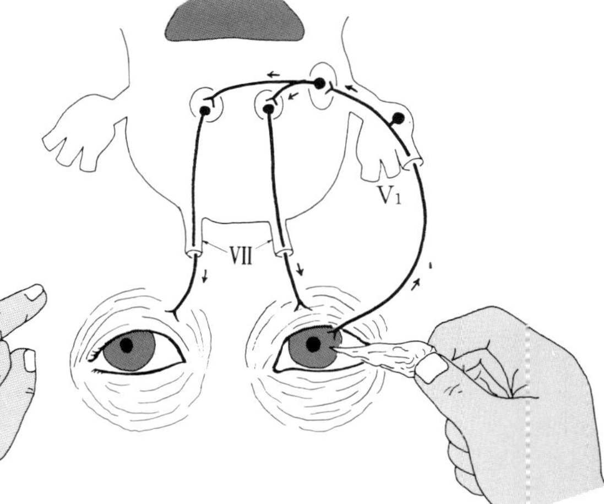

Fig. 109 Testing the corneal reflex and its pathway.
The patient gazes at a point, and the lateral side of cornea is gently stimulated with a wisp of cotton. Care is taken not to stimulate the central area of the cornea, so as not to trigger a visually induced blink reflex.

FACIAL NERVE (VII)

The facial nerve contains motor, sensory and autonomic fibers. Its principal function is to help control movement of the facial muscles. The fibers emerging from the motor nucleus in the pons (110–1) first run posteriorly in the brain stem, then change direction anteriorly to form the internal genu (110–6) and exit the brain stem at the border between the pons and medulla. Subsequently, they enter the internal auditory meatus (110–4) with the eighth cranial nerve (VIII), run in the temporal bone to exit the cranium through the stylomastoid foramen (110–5), and finally supply facial muscles ipsilaterally.

The central pathway of this motor nucleus is different for upper and lower parts of the face. As shown in Fig. 111, muscles in the upper face (orbicularis oculi muscle, etc.) are responsive to bilateral command signals from the cerebral cortex. In contrast, muscles in the lower face (orbicularis oris muscle, etc.) are responsive largely to contralateral commands, like muscles of the upper and lower extremities. As a result, if fibers are damaged peripheral to the nucleus (e.g., the facial nerve itself, 111–B), the ipsilateral side of the face becomes paralyzed both in its upper and lower parts. However, if the damage is more central (e.g., in the internal capsule), muscles in the upper face can still contract (111–A). This distinction helps predict the location of lesions.

Sensory taste fibers supplying the anterior 2/3rds of the tongue project to the solitary nuceus (110–3). Without careful examination, a reduced taste sensation on one side is frequently overlooked. Such a patient tends to sense a rough feeling in one half of the tongue rather than a reduction in taste capacity.

Autonomic fibers project from the superior salivary nucleus (110—2) in the pons to supply the submandibular gland (110–9), sublingual gland (110–10) and lacrimal gland (110–11) to stimulate their secretions*.

Peripheral facial paralysis, Bell's palsy, is caused by strangulation of the swollen nerve (brought on, for example, by viral inflammation in the stylomastoid foramen). If an asymmetry of the patient's face is not obvious at first glance, the disturbance is quickly revealed by asking the patient to close their eyes. Failure to do so results from a dysfunction of the orbicularis oculi muscle. Simultaneously, the eye rotates upwards (controlled by III, IV, VI) and the white of the eye becomes exposed (111-B). This overall disturbance is called lagophthalmus or Bell's phenomenon.

An acoustic neuroma is frequently accompanied by facial nerve palsy. It is more or less expected, because VII and VIII run together in the internal acoustic meatus. Initially, the tumor begins in the internal acoustic meatus, but later it expands towards the cerebello-pontine angle. Finally, the tumor can compress V, IX, X, and XI and the cerebellum (the cerebello-pontine angle syndrome). Therefore, both trigeminal and facial nerve palsy can develop after an operation for acoustic neuroma. It is most important to protect the cornea. If the afferent and efferent pathways of the corneal reflex are disturbed, the eye remains open and dry with reduced lacrimal

---

*The parotid gland has a rather unusual feature. It is well known that operations on this gland can lead to a facial nerve palsy, due to the extensive branching of this nerve as it enters the gland, after emerging from the stylomastoid foramen. Interestingly, the facial nerve does not control secretion of the parotid gland, this being the responsibility of axons of the glossopharyngeal nerve originating in the inferior salivary nucleus.

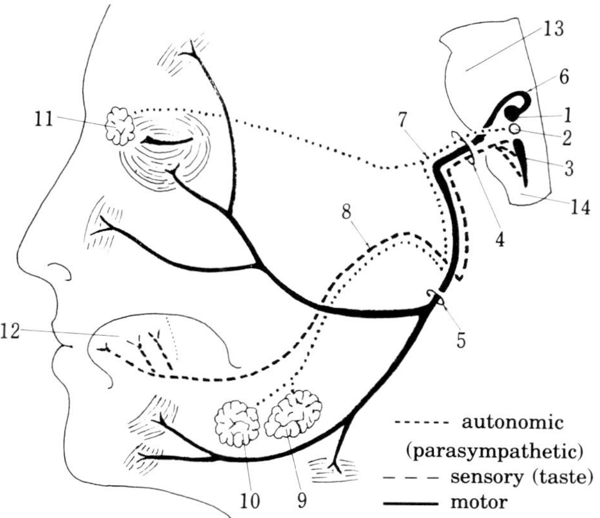

Fig. 110 Distribution of the facial nerve.

1. motor nucleus
2. superior salivary nucleus
3. solitary nucleus
4. internal acoustic meatus
5. stylomastoid foramen
6. genu internum
7. genu externum (geniculate ganglion)
8. chorda tympani nerve
9. submandibular gland
10. sublingual gland
11. lacrimal gland
12. anterior 2/3, taste
13. pons
14. medulla oblongata

secretion and no sensation of pain. There is thus a significant potential for loss of vision. In summary, the most careful attention should be paid to patients with a combined disturbance of trigeminal and facial nerve function.

The Millard-Gubler syndrome, caused by a pontine vascular disorder, has already been described (p. 80).

Hemifacial spasm is a disease which produces involuntary contractions (like spasms) of muscles on one side of the face. In some cases, it has been treated by occipital craniotomy to reduce contact between convoluted blood vessels and the facial nerve.

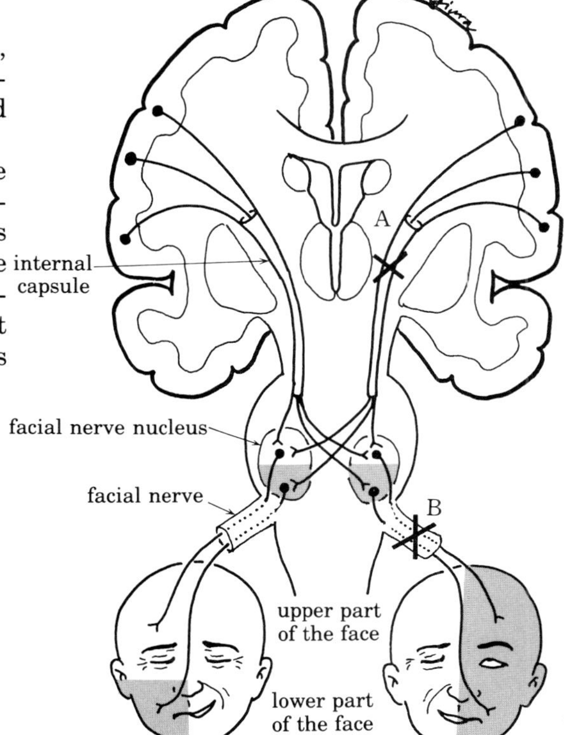

Fig. 111 Facial paralysis.
Note the difference between central (A) and peripheral (B) damage.

STATOACOUSTIC OR AUDITORY NERVE (VIII)

The statoacoustic nerve is divided into the cochlear nerve and the vestibular nerve, both being sensory. The former participates in hearing and the latter in control of equilibrium. From their separate origins in the brain stem, these two nerves run a very short distance together between the pons and medulla, passing through the internal acoustic meatus, to reach the internal ear. Their pathways in the central nervous system are quite different.

The cochlear nerve conducts sound from the organ of Corti in the cochlea (113–1) to the cochlear nucleus in the pons. The central projection is to the lateral lemniscus (113–9), inferior colliculus (113–10), the medial geniculate body (113–11, a part of the thalamus), the auditory radiation and the auditory cortical area (gyrus of Heschl) of the temporal lobe.

The vestibular nerve conducts proprioceptive input from neural epithelium in the ampulla of the semicircular canal, the utricle and the saccule to the vestibular nuclei (113–7) in the medulla and pons. These nuclei have close connections with the cerebellum, spinal cord and eye-movement nuclei. They play an important role in reflex movements required for body balance (Fig. 113).

Symptoms seen in disorders of the cochlear nerve include tinnitus and deafness. These are symptoms of irritation and paralysis, respectively. Tinnitus is a symptom that especially afflicts aged people. Its cause remains unknown and there is no reliable treatment. Deafness, as a concern for the neurosurgeon, is only seen in cases of acoustic neuroma. For accurate localization of deafness, otologic audiometry is necessary. However, a simple hearing test can be used such as shown in Fig. 112. An examiner makes a sound by rubbing together the thumb and index or middle finger. If this sound cannot be heard, Weber's test or Rinne's test with the use of a tuning fork is recommended.

If the vestibular nerve is disturbed, dizziness and nystagmus may occur. Rather than simple problems, these can be complicated and subtle, requiring detailed evaluation by special departments, such as neuro-otology.

Nystagmus is a rhythmic movement of the eye. It is categorized into vertical, horizontal and rotary types, identified by the direction of the rapid-phase of the eye movement. The location of the lesion may be identified by characteristic responses to eye closure, gazing, and change of head position. Nystagmus accompanied by severe vertigo is generally seen in peripheral (internal-ear) disorders.

Although there are many ways of testing vestibular function, a simple bedside technique makes use of a caloric test. Cold water is put in the external acoustic meatus of the supine patient holding a 30– degree head elevation. This produces movement of lymph in the horizontal semi-circular canal which stimulates the vestibular nerve. Consequently, there are induced eye movements. Normally, the nystagmus (rapid phase) is directed toward the opposite side of the cold-water injection and dizziness or vomiting is produced. These reactions disappear early in the course of acoustic neuroma because the tumor develops from the Schwann cells investing the vestibular nerve axons. Meniere's syndrome is well known for its primary symptom of recurrent episodes of dizziness.

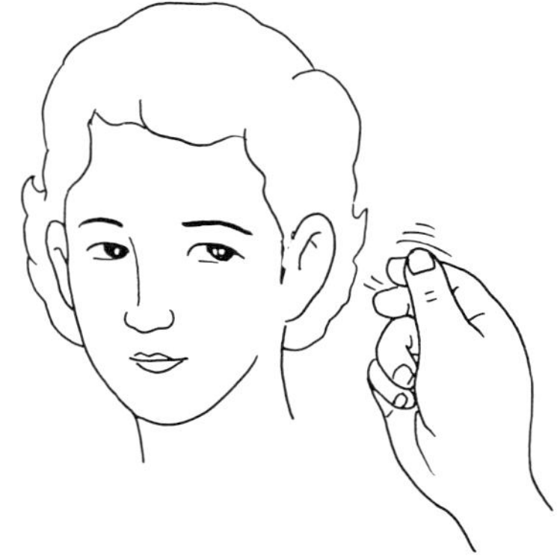

Fig. 112 A simple hearing test.

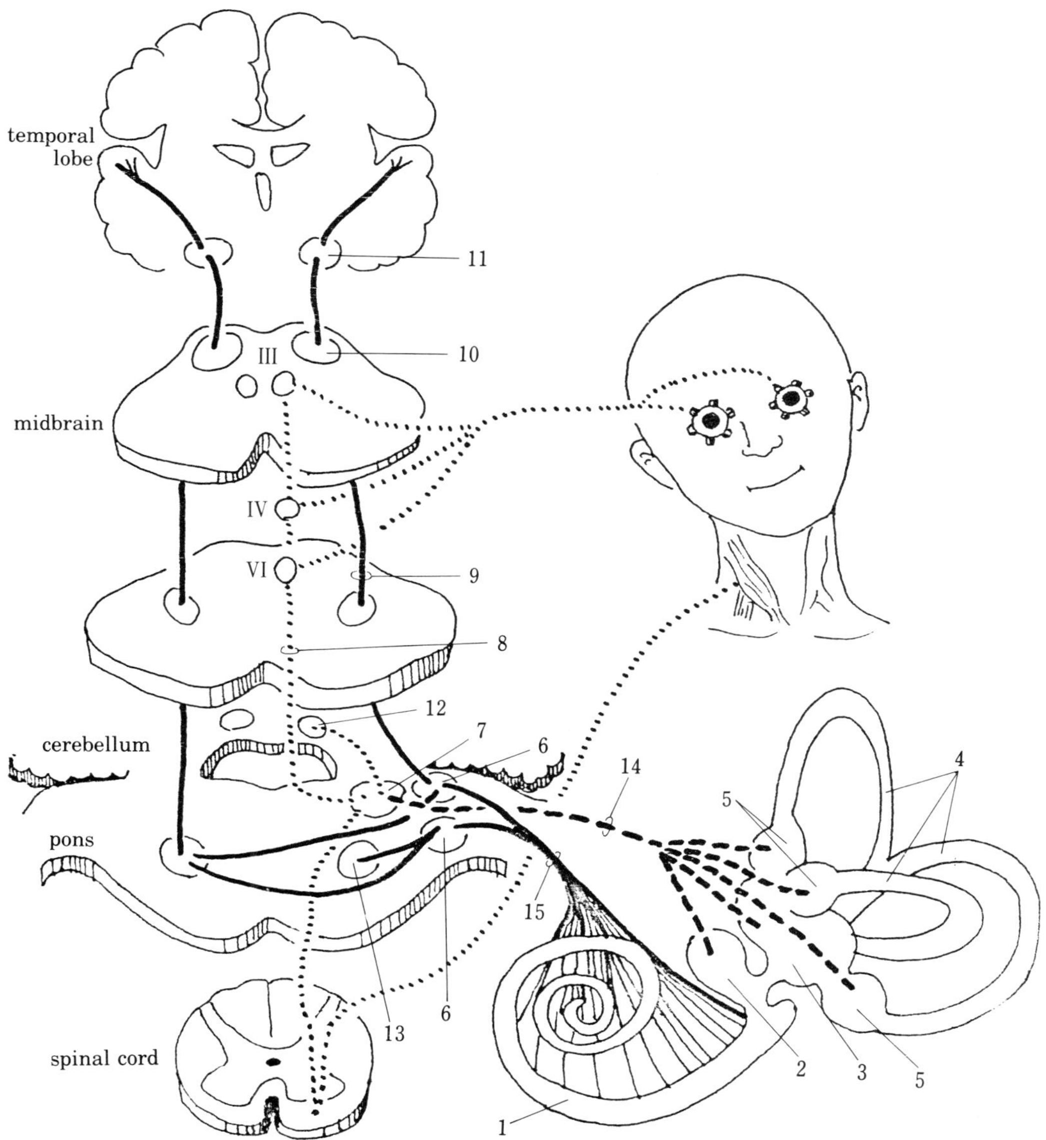

Fig. 113 Pathways of the vestibulo-cochlear nerve.

1. cochlea
2. saccule
3. utricle
4. semicircular canals
5. ampullae
6. cochlear nucleus
7. vestibular nucleus
8. medial longitudinal fasciculus
9. lateral lemniscus
10. inferior colliculus
11. medial geniculate body
12. cerebellar nucleus
13. superior olivary nucleus
14. vestibular nerve
15. cochlear nerve

GLOSSOPHARYNGEAL NERVE (IX)

The glossopharyngeal nerve (IX, Fig. 115) leaves the brain at the superior end of the medulla, and exits the cranium, together with the vagus (X) and the accessory (XI) nerves through the jugular foramen (115–5). The glossopharyngeal, vagus and bulbar rootlets of XI share the same central nucleus and their roles in the control of the larynx and pharynx are somewhat similar.

The sensory supply to the larynx and pharynx is from the glossopharyngeal, while the motor supply is from the vagus and the bulbar rootlets of the accessory nerve.

Sensations in the pharynx, larynx and internal ear (115–12) and sensations (including taste) in the posterior third of the tongue (114, 115–10) result from sensory input conveyed by the glossopharyngeal nerve. This input reaches the solitary nucleus and spinal nucleus of the trigeminal nerve. Subsequent projections are conducted to higher centers. Components of this sensory input are also required for the swallowing reflex, pharyngeal reflexes and reflexes that cause salivary secretion.

Fibers from the carotid sinus (115–7) and carotid body provide the solitary nucleus with information about blood pressure and the partial pressure of blood gases within the carotid artery. Again, subsequent projections are both to higher centers and to local reflexes, the latter being autonomic. Motor fibers in the glossopharyngeal nerve originating in the nucleus ambiguus (115–3) supply the stylopharyngeus muscle (115–6). Its autonomic fibers emerge from the inferior salivary nucleus (115–2) to control parotid gland (115–9) secretion.

A disorder restricted solely to the glossophargyneal nerve is rare, due to its intimate associations, both centrally and peripherally, with the vagus and accessory nerves. The only exception is glossopharyngeal neuralgia. This involves intense pain spasms, like those of trigeminal neuralgia. It was once treated by severing the nerve within the cranium. Now, it is considered sufficient to decompress attached blood vessels around the nerve (after Janetta).

VAGUS NERVE (X)

The close anatomical relationships between the vagus, glossopharyngeal and accessory nerves has already been emphasized. The main function of the vagus nerve is autonomic, with virtually all of these fibers contributing to the parasympathetic system. Vagal parasympathetic fibers originate in the vagus nerve dorsal nucleus, exit the cranium via the jugular foramen, descend along the carotid artery, and then supply various organs, described later. Other vagal fibers controlling movement of the pharynx and larynx (for example, the recurrent laryngeal nerve controlling vocal-cord movement) originate in the nucleus ambiguus (115–3). The vagus contains sensory fibers supplying the external acoustic meatus and dura mater in the posterior cranial fossa. These fibers project to the trigeminal nerve spinal nucleus. If these nuclei are damaged at the level of the medulla, a syndrome called bulbar palsy ensues. It involves functional disorders in nerves IX, X, XI, and XII in which various combinations of disturbances of vocalization, speaking, swallowing, respiration and circulation occur.

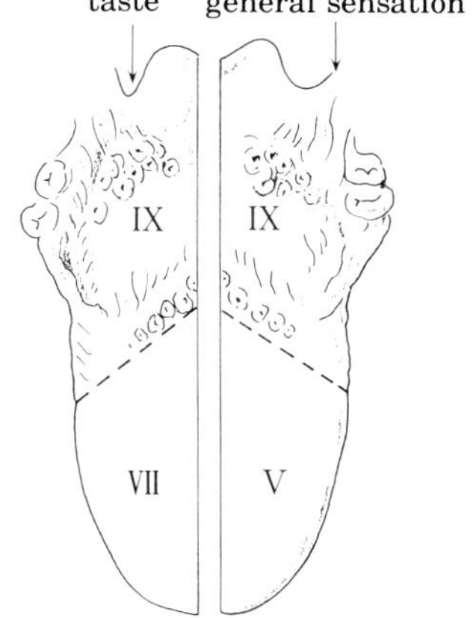

Fig. 114 Sensory innervation of the tongue.

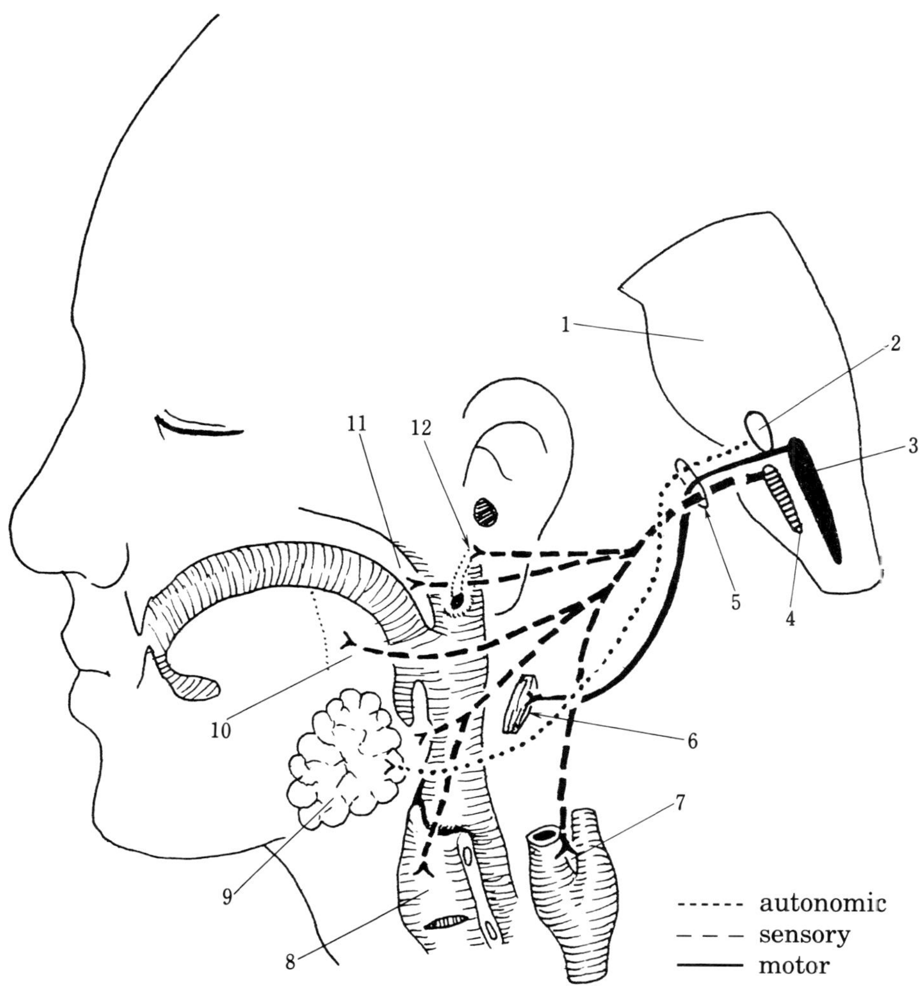

Fig. 115 Distribution of the glossopharyngeal nerve.

1. pons
2. inferior salivary nucleus
3. nucleus ambiguus
4. solitary nucleus
5. jugular foramen
6. stylopharyngeus muscle
7. carotid sinus
8. larynx
9. parotid gland
10. posterior 1/3rd of tongue (taste and sensory)
11. soft palate
12. middle ear

ACCESSORY NERVE (XI)

This is virtually a pure motor nerve divided into two roots: a cranial one emerging from the medulla and a spinal one from the first to the sixth segment of the cervical cord. The cranial root (medullary portion, 117–5) originates in the nucleus ambiguus (117–2), runs a short distance as the independent accessory nerve (the so-called bulbar rootlets), and then merges into the vagus nerve (117–X) just outside the cranium. This root controls movements of the pharynx and larynx.

The spinal portion (117–6) of the accessory nerve exits into the subarachnoid space along with the anterior roots of the spinal nerves from the anterior horn of the first to the fifth or sixth cervical segments of the cord. This route is a little unusual because it ascends in the subarachnoid space into the cranium through the foramen

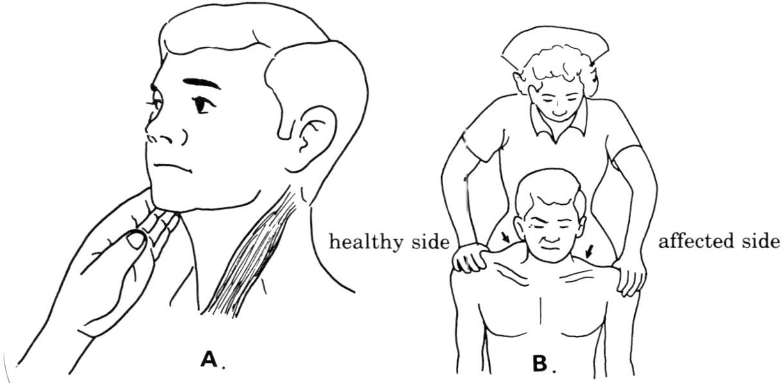

Fig. 116 An accessory nerve test.

A. The left sternocleidomastoid muscle rotates the head to the right. The examiner provides resistance to the movement.
B. Reduced muscle force of the trapezius muscle on the left side.

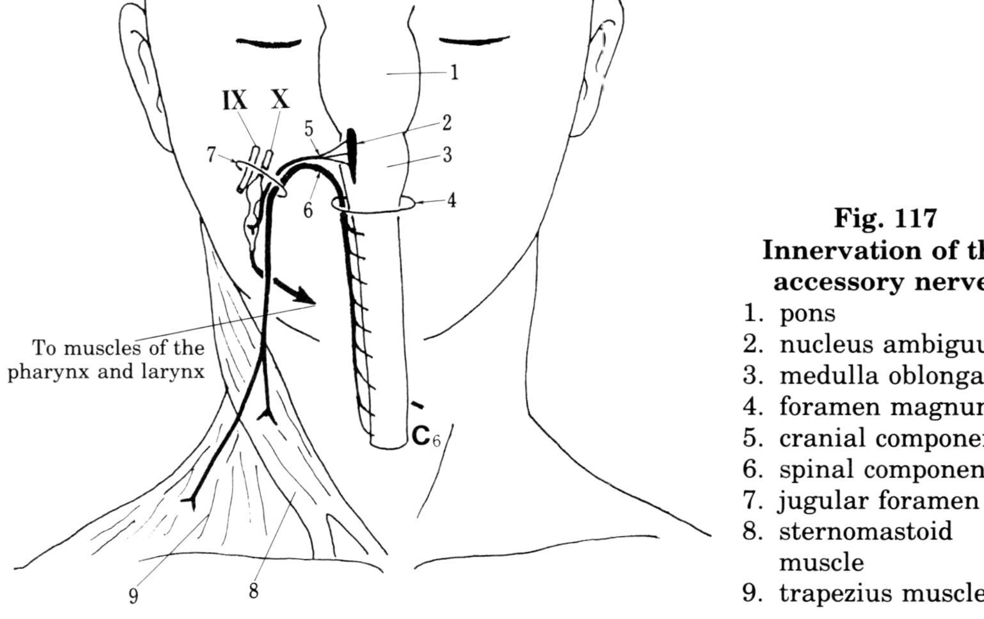

Fig. 117 Innervation of the accessory nerve.

1. pons
2. nucleus ambiguus
3. medulla oblongata
4. foramen magnum
5. cranial component
6. spinal component
7. jugular foramen
8. sternomastoid muscle
9. trapezius muscle

magnum (117–4), before exiting the cranium again through the jugular foramen (117–7) to supply the sternocleidomastoid (117–8) and trapezius (117–9) muscles.

The accessory nerve is rarely disturbed independently, but is usually compromised together with nerves IX, X or XII. Similarly, its cranial root is rarely damaged independently. In the case of a disorder of the spinal root, the patient can neither rotate the head to the contralateral side (a function of the sternocleidomastoid muscle, 116–A) nor elevate the shoulder on the affected side (trapezius muscle, 116–B).

HYPOGLOSSAL NERVE (XII)

This is a pure motor nerve (at least in adult) which totally controls movements of the tongue. Fibers from the hypoglossal nucleus (119–1) exit the medulla into the hypoglossal canal lateral to the foramen magnum (119–2) and then leave the cranium to supply various muscles. Since innervation from the hypoglossal nucleus is predominantly ipsilateral, deviation of the tongue is readily seen during central or supranuclear palsy. Independent palsy of the hypoglossal nerve is rarely seen. Palsy can be clearly detected by noting tongue movements. If there is a peripheral disorder, the tongue on the paralyzed side cannot be extended. It is forced to the affected side by the contralateral (healthy) side (Fig. 118). If the palsy occurs centrally, deviation of the tongue is directed toward the contralateral side of the lesion, because of the central crossing of supranuclear fibers.

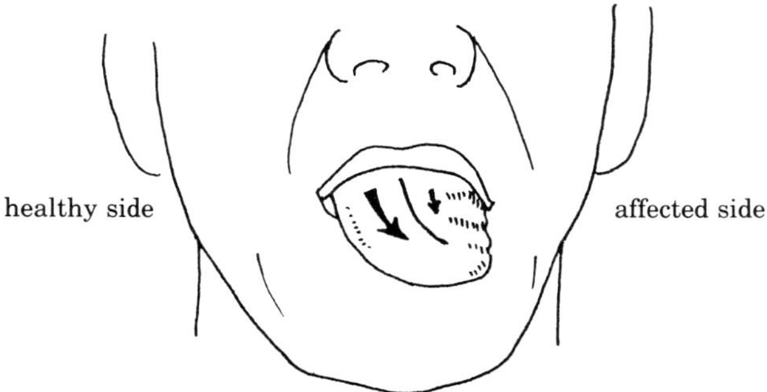

Fig. 118 Peripheral hypoglossal paralysis.

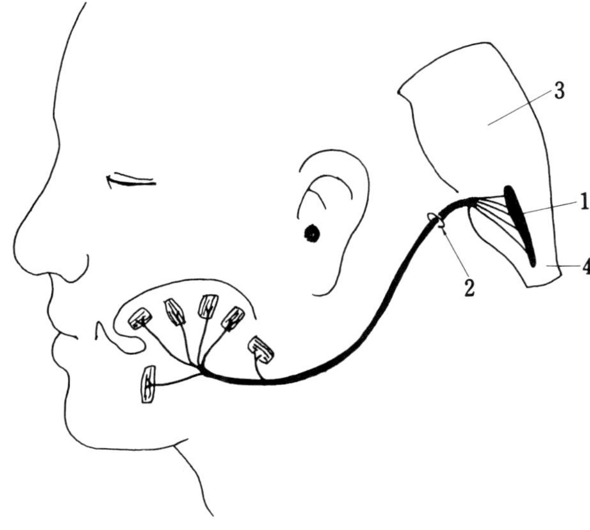

Fig. 119 Distribution of the hypoglossal nerve.

1. hypoglossal nucleus
2. hypoglossal canal
3. pons
4. medulla oblongata

7. AUTONOMIC NERVOUS SYSTEM

The autonomic nervous system, supplying cardiac and smooth muscle and glandular tissue, subconsciously controls the internal status of the body to provide appropriate changes to both internal and external stimuli.

This system is divided into two components, the sympathetic and the parasympathetic, with generally opposing functions. Table 11 lists these functions for selected organs. This table is easily understood if one remembers that the sympathetic system functions under conditions of heavy stress or emergency to mobilize the organism to act quickly and forcefully. In contrast, the parasympathetic system has a restorative effect on a body, including voiding actions. To appreciate sympathetic actions, imagine a human confronting a ferocious animal, like a lion. To escape rapidly, the muscles must be activated optimally. Blood supply to these muscles is also optimized by vessel dilation. The heart begins to beat strongly and the coronary arteries also dilate to optimize the blood supply to the heart. Concomitantly, arteries supplying the skin and viscera constrict, because these organs need little blood during exercise. Churning activity of the stomach and intestines is also reduced as well as the secretion of glands. Augmented cardiac output would be ineffective without increased oxygen in the blood, so the bronchi dilate. Dilation of the pupil is needed to enhance visual input during high-speed flight. Piloerection is evident and increased sweating is needed to augment heat loss from the hard-working body.

As for parasympathetic actions, imagine how the above-mentioned organs would work during dinner in a pleasant family atmosphere!

It is convenient to think of the hypothalamus as the center for autonomic control. This structure's descending projections through the brain stem are complex and concentrated largely in the reticular formation.

Peripheral autonomic nerves consist of motor (efferent) fibers, and sensory (afferent) fibers. The cell bodies of the sensory axons are located in the spinal ganglia. Many of these sensory fibers conduct location-poor information about pain and GI disturbances to the central nervous system. Other sensory fibers contribute input required for a wide variety of autonomic reflexes.

The cell bodies of sympathetic motor axons are located in the lateral horn of the spinal gray matter extending from the upper thoracic cord to the upper part of the lumbar cord. They emerge from the spinal cord through the anterior root, then leave the spinal nerve after passing through the intervertebral foramen, to enter a sympathetic ganglion (120–2, 3). Longitudinally connected groups of sympathetic ganglia on both sides of the spinal column are called sympathetic trunks (120–1). Sympathetic fibers do not emerge from cervical or sacral segments of the spinal cord, but sympathetic ganglia are found at cervical and sacral levels. The stellate ganglion (120–2), at the lowest cervical level, is particularly prominent. Besides these sympathetic trunk ganglia, there are some others in the abdominal cavity (120–4).

Table 11. FUNCTIONS OF THE SYMPATHETIC AND PARASYMPATHETIC SYSTEMS

	SYMPATHETIC	PARASYMPATHETIC
heart rate	↑	↓
bronchi	dilation	constriction
coronary arteries	dilation	→
arteries in skeletal muscles	dilation	→
blood vessels in the skin and viscera	constriction	dilation
pupils	dilation	constriction
digestive organs (movement, secretion)	decreased	increased
piloerector muscles	stimulated	—
sweat glands	stimulated	—

Fibers from all the sympathetic ganglia are distributed to visceral organs, blood vessels, glands, the eyes and so on. The cell bodies of parasympathetic axons are located in several brain stem nuclei including the Edinger-Westphal nucleus (120–5), the superior and inferior salivatory nuclei (120–6) and the dorsal nucleus of the vagus nerve (120–7), and in the lateral horn of the sacral cord (120–S). It has been mentioned that fibers from the Edinger-Westphal nucleus contribute to the oculomotor nerve (120–III), those from the superior and inferior salivatory nucleus to the facial nerve (120–VII) and those from the dorsal nucleus of the vagus to the vagus nerve.

Fibers from the central nervous system to all autonomic ganglia are called preganglionic fibers, and those from the ganglia to the target organs are called postganglionic fibers. Acetylcholine is the chemical transmitter secreted at all autonomic nerve endings except sympathetic postganglionic fibers which secrete norepinephrine.

Horner's syndrome is a well-known disorder of cervical sympathetic axons. Its symptoms include enophthalmos, miosis, ptosis and flushing of the face on the affected side. It is sometimes necessary to distinguish this condition from oculomotor nerve palsy. This judgement is aided by noting that the latter condition involves a more severe ptosis and the pupil malfunction is mydriasis, rather than miosis.

As for surgical intervention in the autonomic nervous system, a sympathetic ganglionectomy may be carried out to dilate blood vessels in ischemic diseases such as reflex sympathetic dystrophy.

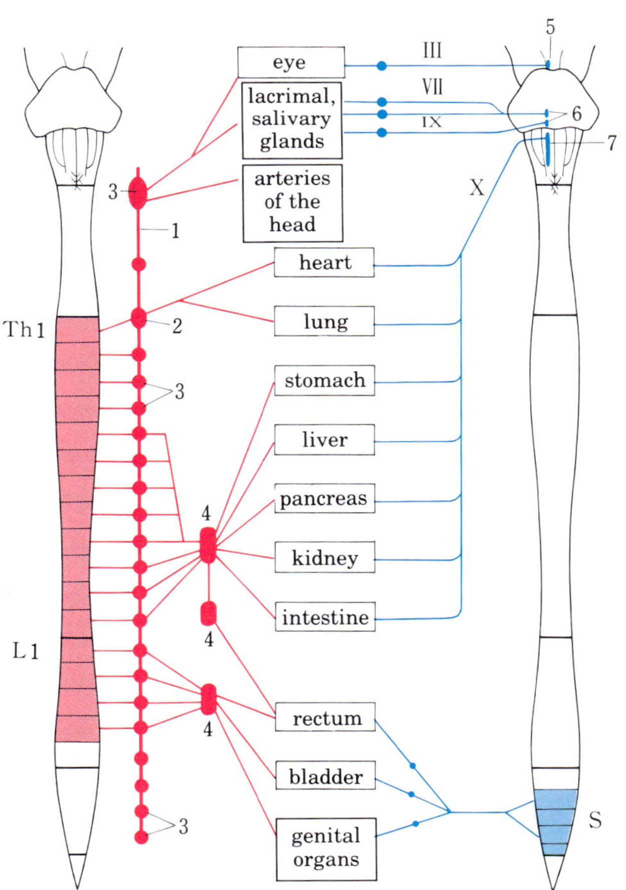

1. sympathetic trunk
2. stellate ganglion
3. sympathetic ganglia
4. celiac ganglion
5. Edinger-Westphal nucleus
6. superior and inferior salivary nuclei
7. dorsal nucleus of the vagus nerve

III. oculomotor nerve
VII. facial nerve
IX. glossopharyngeal nerve
X. vagus nerve

Fig. 120 Sympathetic and parasympathetic structures (after Villinger and Ludwig).

8. MAJOR CENTRAL PATHWAYS

PYRAMIDAL TRACT

When this term is used for motor pathways crossing at or below the pyramids in the medulla, it involves pathways controlling voluntary movement of the upper and lower extremities. However, the term is sometimes used in a wider sense, as in this textbook, to represent most of the motor pathways (including those within cranial nerves) which control voluntary movement.

The original (first-order) neurons whose fibers form the pyramidal tract are located in the motor area of the frontal lobe (61–4, 121). The tract forms in this area and projects downwards through the posterior limb of the internal capsule (121–1). Then, it passes through the cerebral peduncle (121–2), the ventral pons and the pyramids of the medulla (121–3), below which, most of the tract's axons cross the midline (pyramidal decussation, 121–4) to enter the lateral funiculus and descend to finally terminate on or near the spinal anterior horn cells supplying the various body parts.

The cranial nerves control voluntary movements of the eye (oculomotor 121–III, trochlear 121–IV, abducens 121–VI), the face (facial 121–VII), the larynx (glossopharyngeal 121–IX, vagus 121–X), the neck (accessory 121–XI) and the tongue (hypoglossal 121–XII). Pyramidal tract innervation of these nuclei is largely by way of axons which cross the midline just above the supplied nucleus. Except for neurons supplying lower face muscles and occasionally the tongue, there is also a small uncrossed pyramidal tract innervation. As a result, central damage of the pyramidal tract on one side does not always result in a clear-cut contralateral disorder of movements controlled by the cranial nerves.

The pyramidal tract occupies a wide area of the cortex and subcortex. It becomes progressively narrower as it descends into the internal capsule, pons, medulla and spinal cord. For a similarly sized lesion, the more caudal the location, the wider the area of peripheral motor paralysis.

Table 12. PARALYSIS AS A FUNCTION OF LESION LOCATION

lesion	symptom
cerebral cortex or subcortex	monoplegia (one extremity)
internal capsule-cerebral peduncle	hemiplegia + paralysis in lower face
pons	hemiplegia + paralysis in opposite upper and lower face
lower pons (or medulla)	hemiplegia (without facial paralysis)
cervical cord	quadriplegia
thoracic cord (or lower)	paraplegia (lower extremities)

EXTRAPYRAMIDAL SYSTEM

This is a general term for all descending motor pathways except the pyramidal tract. Most of this system, functioning subconsciously, provides the motor support required for smooth voluntary movement. For example, when the pyramidal system commands flexion of the arm, the extrapyramidal system comes into play to see that all other relevant muscles have appropriate activity levels for the arm flexion to achieve its purpose. Without such supportive extrapyramidal action, skillful movements of the arms and legs would not be possible.

Brain structures contributing axons to the extrapyramidal system include the frontal lobe (except for area 4), basal ganglia, red nucleus and substantia nigra, cerebellum, vestibular nuclei and reticular formation in the brain stem. These centers have complex interconnections and interactions, their details are far from resolved.

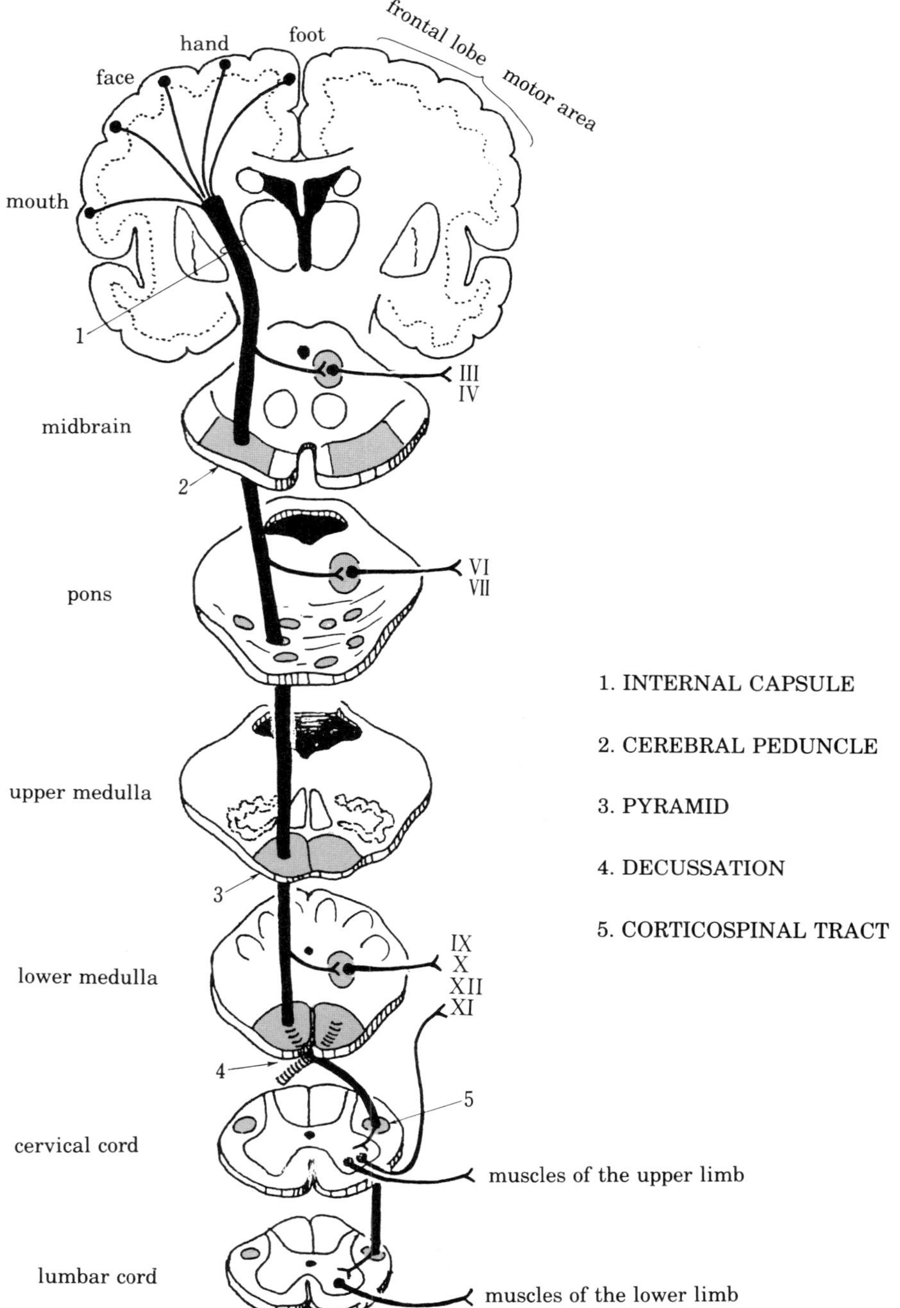

Fig. 121 The pyramidal tract.
A schematic diagram of the pyramidal tract which controls voluntary movements. Cranial-nerve nuclei and pathways are simplified here. Except for a part of VII and XII, there is also a small uncrossed pyramidal tract invervation to all the cranial nerve nuclei.

MOTOR PATHWAY DISORDERS AND THEIR SYMPTOMS

Lesions of the pyramidal tract cause disorders of voluntary movement. If the patient cannot move the arms and legs voluntarily, the deficit is called paralysis. It is classified not only by the location of the peripheral deficit, such as monoplegia and hemiplegia (viz. Table 12), but also by the location of damaged neurons, as in central or peripheral paralysis.

Peripheral paralysis occurs when damage is to motoneurons (and neighboring interneurons) of the brain stem and spinal cord. This paralysis is termed flaccid, meaning that muscle tone and tendon reflexes are greatly reduced or absent; atrophy and fasciculations occur and even pathological reflexes cannot be elicited.

On the other hand, spastic paralysis is seen in the case of a central paralysis caused by lesions in more centrally located neurons including those contributing axons to the pyramidal and extrapyramidal tracts. In this case, the tone of affected muscles increases to display spasticity and/or rigidity. Tendon reflexes are hyperactive, and clonus or other pathological reflexes may be present. Muscle atrophy is usually not found except for a secondary atrophy due to disuse of the extremities. Although there are many ways to demonstrate pathological reflexes in the extremities, testing should always include a Hoffmann reflex (122–b) in the fingers and a Babinski reflex (122–a) in the foot.

Involuntary-movement syndromes due to extrapyramidal lesions have already been presented. However, more should be said about abnormal muscle tonus, brought about by disorders of the pyramidal and extrapyramidal tracts.

Spasticity is usually seen in the case of pyramidal tract disorders (123–a). It is revealed when the examiner begins to move the patient's hand or foot. First, a strong resistance is encountered to passive movement. Then, this resistance subsides rapidly. This resistance pattern is similar to that of a clasp-knife being opened. Hence,

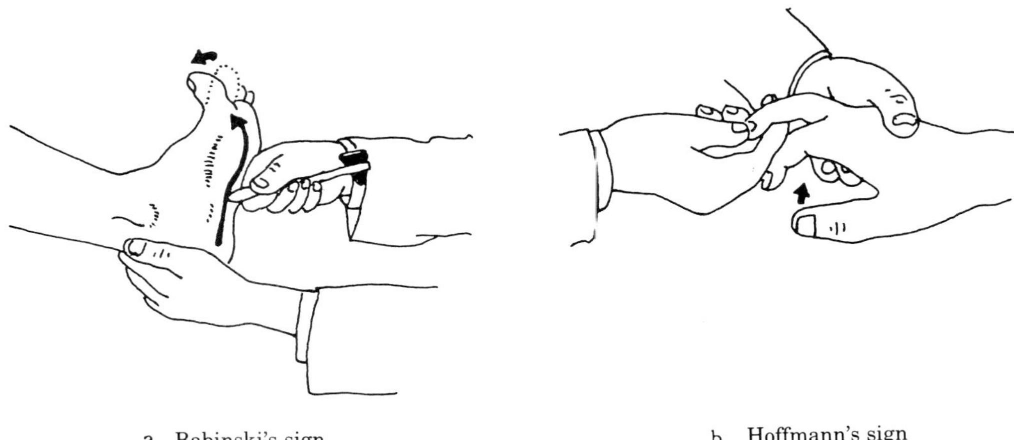

a. Babinski's sign　　b. Hoffmann's sign

Fig. 122 Examination of a representative pathological reflex.

a. When the sole is stroked with a sharp object, from the outer border of the heel upwards, the great toe extends dorsally and the other toes spread like a fan (the Babinski reflex).

b. When the tip of the middle finger is flipped, a brisk flexion and adduction of the thumb is observed (the Hoffmann reflex).

this is called the clasp-knife phenomenon.

Another form of increased muscle tonus is called rigidity. It results from diseases or damage to the extrapyramidal system. From the beginning to the end of a passive movement two kinds of rigidity are seen: the lead-pipe phenomenon (123–b) in which continuous resistance can be felt and the cog-wheel phenomenon (123–c) in which a discontinuous resistance is present.

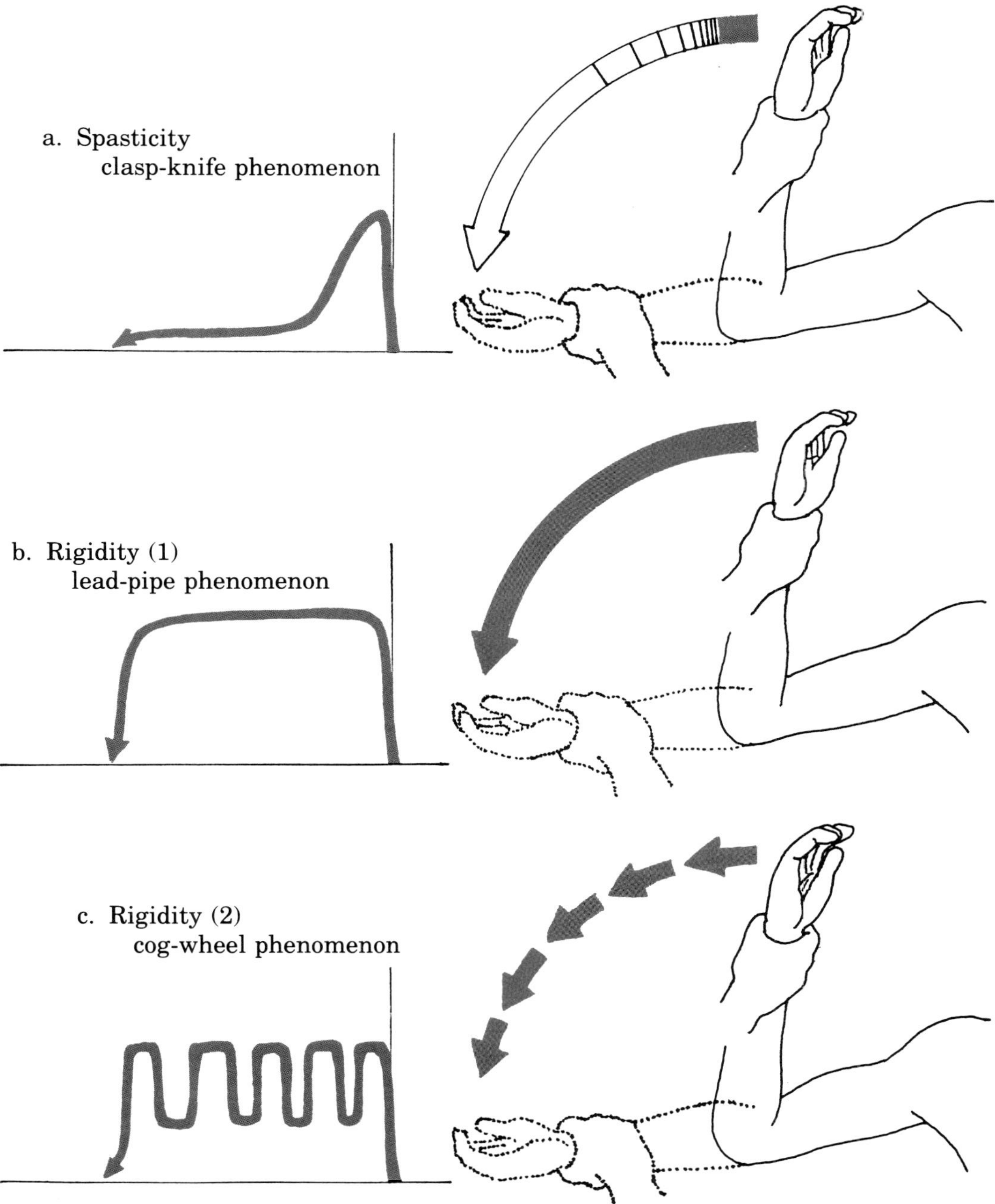

Fig. 123 Disorders of muscle tonus

PAIN-TEMPERATURE AND PROPRIOCEPTIVE PATHWAYS

The cell bodies of primary neurons conducting pain and temperature information are located in the spinal ganglia (124–1). Their central axonal projections through the posterior spinal roots are to second-order neurons in the posterior horn (124–2). Subsequent projections immediately cross the midline and ascend in the lateral funiculus (124–3) and brain stem to reach the thalamus (124–5). This pathway is called the spinothalamic tract (124–4).

Although the cell bodies of the primary sensory neurons conducting proprioceptive information (pressure, joint position, vibration, etc.) are also located in spinal ganglia, their central axonal projections are quite different to those of pain-temperature axons. One collateral of each proprioceptive axon immediately enters the ipsilateral posterior funiculus (dorsal column pathway). Some of these ascend to the nucleus gracilis (125—3) and nucleus cuneatus (125–4) in the lower medulla. However, most posterior funiculus axons are relatively short, with several neurons being required to bring proprioceptive information to the gracile and cuneate nuclei. Subsequent projections from these nuclei cross the midline in the medulla and ascend in the brain stem as part of the medial lemniscus (125–5) which projects to the thalamus (125–6).

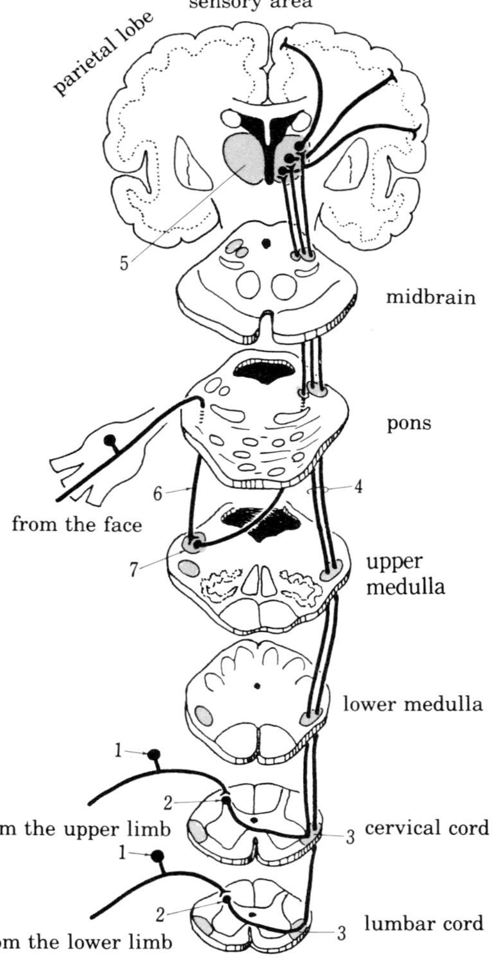

Fig. 124 The pathways for pain and temperature.

Fibers entering the spinal cord through the dorsal root excite second-order neurons whose axons cross to the contralateral side. The pain-temperature pathway from the face (via the trigeminal nerve) is also shown.

1. dorsal root ganglia
2. second-order neurons in the posterior horn
3. lateral funiculus
4. spinothalamic tract
5. thalamus
6. spinal tract of the trigeminal nerve
7. spinal nucleus of the trigeminal nerve

From the description above, it is obvious that disorders of pain-temperature and proprioception can help when deciding on the site (side) of a spinal lesion. Interestingly, disorders of tactile sensation are not so helpful, because the relevant central pathways are more complex before joining the medial lemniscal system. Sensory information about pain-temperature, proprioception and touch is relayed to third and subsequent-order neurons in the thalamus. Their axons ascend through the posterior limb of the internal capsule to reach relevant sensory areas (61–1, 2, 3) in the parietal lobe.

Abnormalities of sensation occur with lesions to these various routes. The most frequent disease is hemihypoesthesia or paresthesia as a sequela of cerebrovascular disorders in the brain. In particular, an abnormal sensation or pain in the upper and lower extremities after a vascular accident in the thalamus is well known (Dejerine-Roussy syndrome). The neurosurgical issue in these cases is the amelioration of the pain. Surgical methods available which can be used to relieve pain in other areas and due to other causes may include: antero-lateral cordotomy to interrupt the pain pathway, electrical stimulation of the thalamus or central gray matter to evoke secretion of endorphins and electrical stimulation of various other parts of the central or peripheral nervous system to block pain perception.

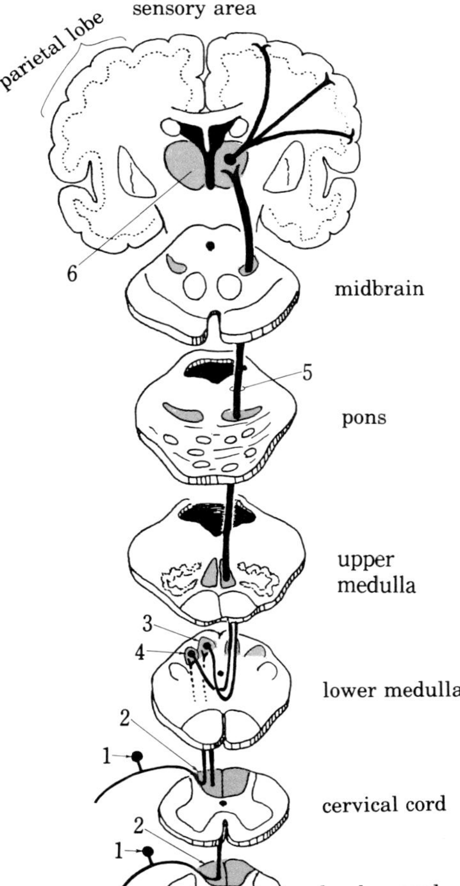

Fig. 125 Pathways for proprioception. Fibers entering through the dorsal root contribute directly to the ipsilateral dorsal column. The second-order medullary neuron's axon crosses the midline to form the medial lemniscus. Not shown are the many dorsal column axons that synapse frequently before reaching the dorsal column nuclei.

1. dorsal root ganglia
2. posterior funiculus
3. nucleus gracilis
4. nucleus cuneatus
5. medial lemniscus
6. thalamus

II. PATHOLOGICAL PHYSIOLOGY

1. INCREASED INTRACRANIAL PRESSURE

INTRACRANIAL PRESSURE (ICP)

It is no exaggeration to state that a major concern of most neurosurgeons is the early detection of increased ICP. Awareness of it is essential when treating neurosurgical diseases. The skull is designed to protect the brain from external injury. However, if ICP rises due to an intracranial disturbance, the skull subjects the brain tissue to the full impact of this pressure, and self-destruction becomes an issue.

Within the cranium, the brain substance, blood and cerebrospinal fluid are maintained in relatively fixed proportions (Figs. 126, 127). The ICP is usually kept near 100–150mm H_2O (10mm Hg). If the volume of a normal intracranial component increases or a pathological material is added (e.g., hematoma, tumor), the ICP will increase. If the volume decreases, ICP will decrease. When considering ICP, it is helpful to evaluate increases and decreases of each component separately. However, clinical problems most frequently involve only increases in ICP. Decreases are only seen in decreased cerebrospinal fluid syndrome, usually brought on by lumbar puncture.

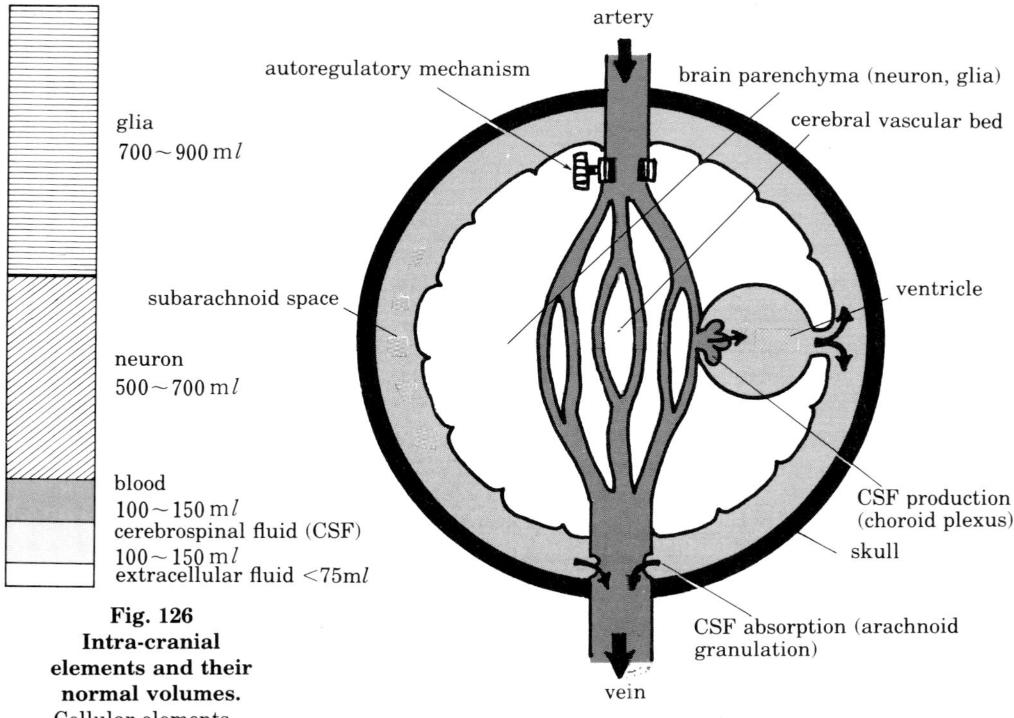

Fig. 126 Intra-cranial elements and their normal volumes. Cellular elements occupying most of these components are rather constant except in the case of edema. Volume changes are normally seen mainly in the blood and cerebrospinal fluid.

Fig. 127 A schematic diagram of the contents of the cranium. Study of these structures gives insight into the mechanisms of increased intracranial pressure.

BRAIN EDEMA—INCREASED VOLUME OF BRAIN SUBSTANCE

The volume of brain substance increases during brain edema. The mechanisms underlying this problem are still controversial, but a disturbance of the blood-brain barrier (BBB) is usually involved.

When a pigment like trypan blue is injected in the blood, almost all the tissues of the body are stained. However, the brain and spinal cord are not normally stained except for the choroid plexus, pineal body and hypophysis. This suggests that a special boundary exists between the blood and the brain. It is called the blood-brain barrier.

The BBB is more than an anatomical structure. The endothelial cells of the brain's capillaries are connected to each other by tight junctions (128–1) unlike other parts of the body through which molecules can more easily pass. There are no pericapillary spaces in the brain, like those in other parts of the body. Instead, basement membranes (128–2, 130) and astrocytic processes (endfeet) densely surround the capillaries (128–3). Again, these characteristics are markedly different from structures near capillaries in other parts of the body. Thus, there is indeed a structural basis for the BBB, within which additional physiological mechanisms are incorporated.

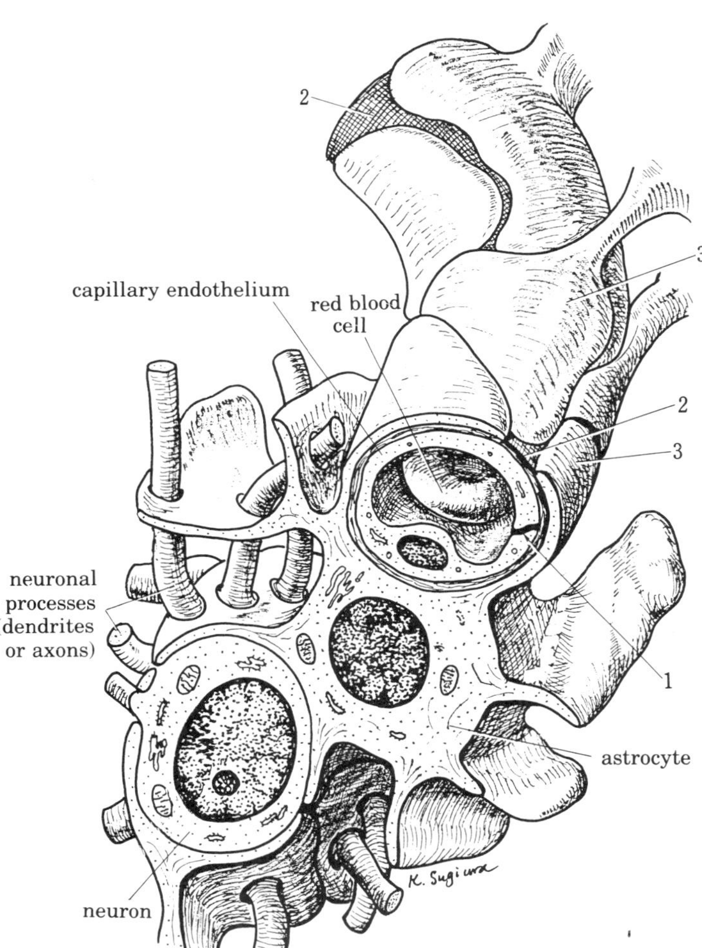

1. capillary tight junction
2. basement membrane
3. astrocyte foot process

Fig. 128 Capillaries and astrocytes in the brain - the blood-brain barrier (after R.V. Kristic).

In brain edema, fluid leaked from the blood stays in or between cells in the brain. In pathological situations it is quite common (Figs. 129, 130). As described later, the term "brain swelling" has a similar meaning. However, it should be distinguished from edema because it is caused by expansion of the vascular bed.

Brain edema is divided into cytotoxic and vasogenic types, based on their separate etiologies. But, to varying degrees, they often occur together.

Cytotoxic edema typically occurs when a metabolic toxin such as methyl tin enters the body. The mechanism underlying this type of edema is a loss of the normal function of the cell membrane. However, at the outset, the BBB is not necessarily compromised. Rather, the hyperpermeability caused by the toxin first causes the cell body to swell with an abnormal intake of the fluid. At this stage, the intercellular space is somewhat reduced, due to the movement of fluid intracellularly. Later, the entire brain substance expands due to the entrance of fluid from the vascular bed. In contrast, vasogenic edema is a primary concern in almost all the clinical conditions associated with trauma, neurosurgical intervention, brain tumor and inflammation. It develops from a disruption of the BBB, causing protein-rich fluid to enter from the vascular bed into the intercellular space, and to infiltrate the white matter via an osmotic gradient. In summary, an increased intercellular space is quite pronounced at the beginning of this type of edema, but as it progresses the cells themselves may become swollen and functionless (Fig. 130).

Blood pressure plays an important role in the edematous process. Increasing pressure speeds and decreasing pressure slows the progress of edema, especially the vasogenic type. Osmotic pressure is also a key factor. The ingestion of water exacerbates edema. On the other hand, drugs which increase osmotic pressure (e.g., mannitol) reduce and delay its progress.

More emphasis should be placed on the prevention of brain edema, rather than its treatment. To this end, mannitol as an osmotic pressure diuretic and steroids are particularly useful.

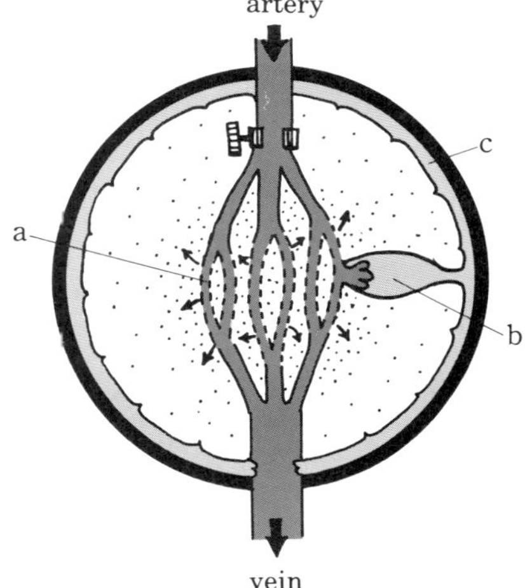

Fig. 129 Brain edema schematic.
When the blood-brain barrier is compromised, the vascular compartment leaks into brain tissue (arrows). A compensatory reduction of the ventricles and subarachnoid space then occurs.

A. normal

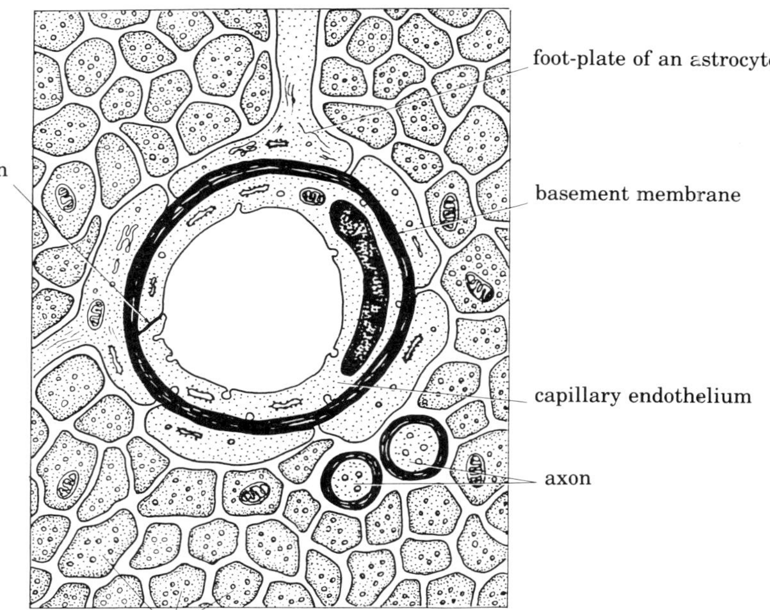

B. abnormal (edema)

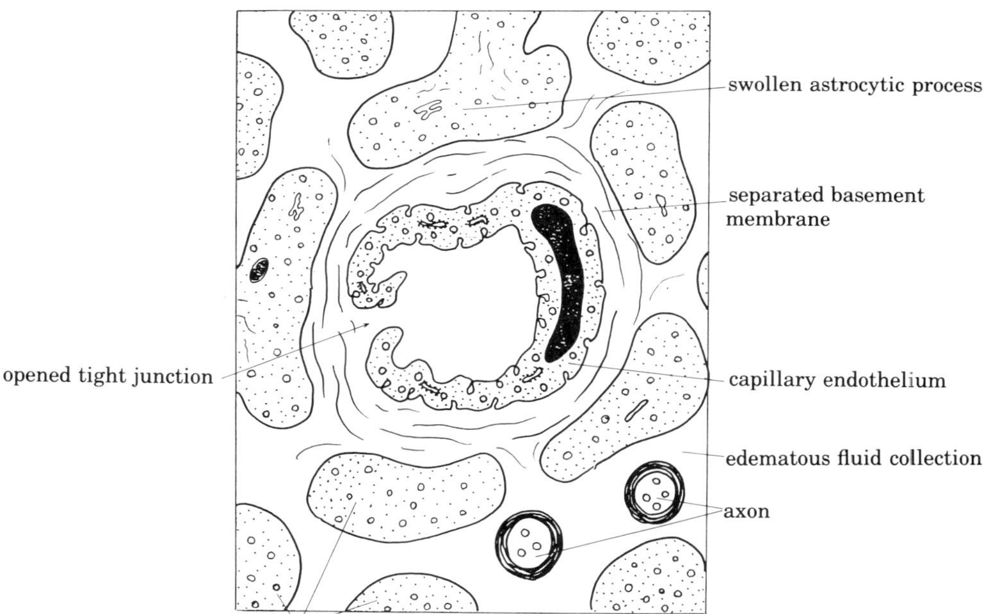

Fig. 130 A microscopic view of brain edema.
Note the disturbance of structural organization normally associated with the capillary and its surrounding basement membrane. The cell body swells and the intercellular space increases remarkably.

HYDROCEPHALUS—THE EXPANSION OF CEREBROSPINAL FLUID

Cerebrospinal fluid (CSF) is secreted mainly by the papillae of the choroid plexus in the ventricles (Fig. 42) and is absorbed after completing its circulation via the superior sagittal sinus. The causes of increased CSF within the cranium are thought to be increases in CSF secretion and decreases in CSF absorption. However, the former disturbance is very rare (e.g. papilloma of the choroid plexus). Rather, a pathological increase in the volume of intracranial CSF is invariably due to a disturbance in absorption, brought on by closure or constriction of a CSF pathway (Fig. 131). If the ventricles expand in hydrocephalus, intracerebral forces increase and the function of the brain is endangered not only by the pressure increase but also by the subsequent distortion of brain parenchyma.

Surgical treatment is usually needed for hydrocephalus. Ventricular drainage can be carried out on a temporary basis, but a ventriculo-peritoneal (VP) shunt or a ventriculo-atrial (VA) shunt should be considered for definitive treatment of chronic cases. After dealing with acute hemorrhage, inflammation or trauma within the cranium, it is important to eliminate the possibility of hydrocephalus as a secondary complication. The surgical technique is easy and effective, but, if it is not timely, an irreversible cerebral disorder will occur.

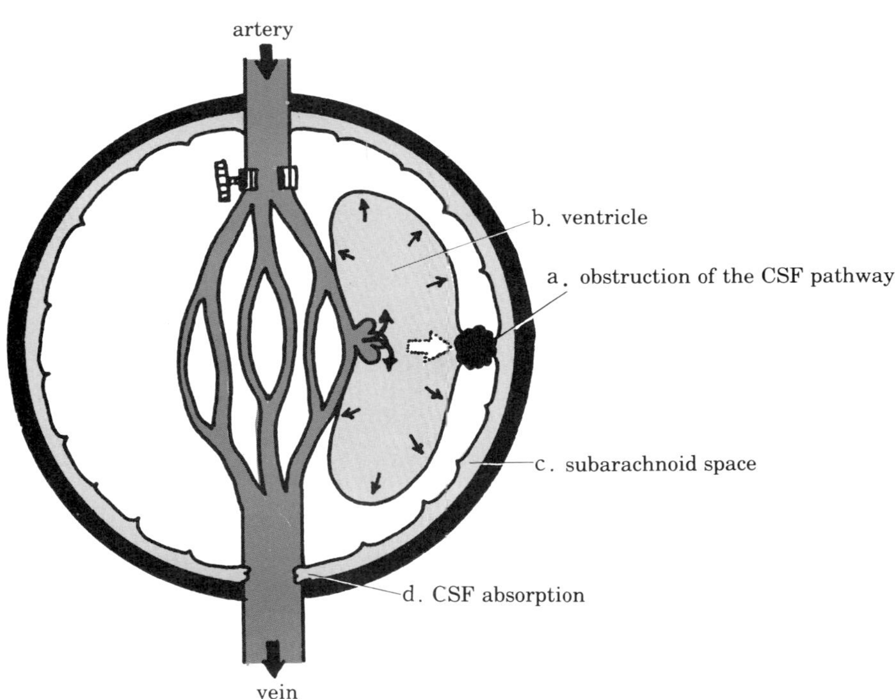

Fig. 131 Hydrocephalus.

This diagram of a non-communicating hydrocephalus shows expansion of a ventricle (b) caused by tumor blockage (a). Stenosis or obstruction of the subarachnoid space (c) and/or arachnoid granulations (d) may also cause ventricular enlargement.

BRAIN SWELLING—INCREASED BLOOD VOLUME

Undoubtedly, the blood volume is the most rapidly adjustable intracranial component available for the regulation of pressure within the cranium. During brain swelling, increased blood volume occurs in the vascular bed in one of two forms: venous system congestion (132—b) or arterial system hyperemia (132—a).

There is no valve between cranial veins and the superior vena cava. Therefore, increased intrathoracic pressure (associated with choking, coughing, convulsions) brings on high venous pressure which disturbs venous drainage from the brain and causes increased intracranial pressure. Excessive neck flexion or pressure applied to the neck is also followed by increased intracranial pressure due to blood flow disturbances in the jugular veins. Occasionally, ice is packed on the neck of a patient with cranial trauma. This is not necessarily a sound treatment because a subsequently applied Queckenstedt test* may bring on an unexpected increase in intracranial pressure due to neck compression. When the pressure is measured during a lumbar puncture, the neck should be placed in a relaxed position to obviate a false pressure reading.

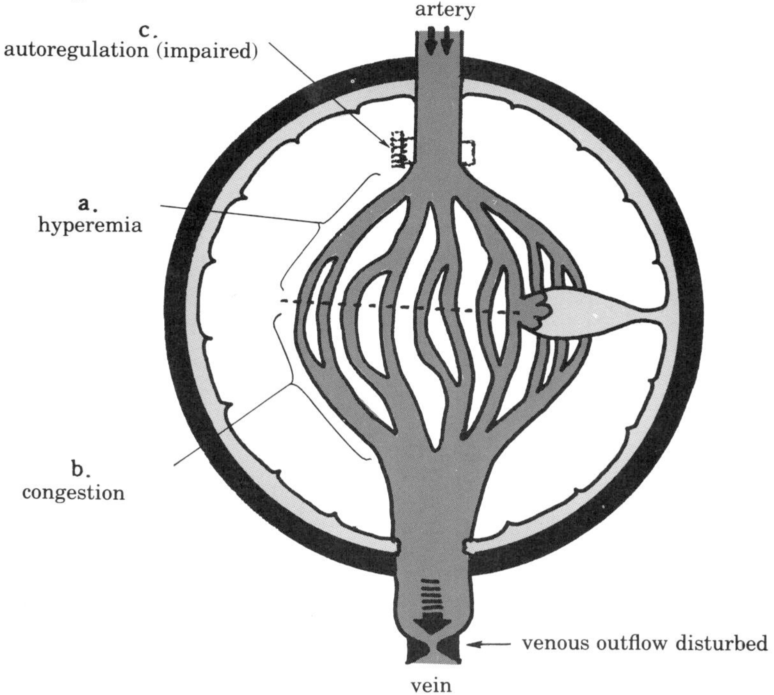

Fig. 132 Brain swelling.

Hyperemia and congestion are caused by arterial dilation or an obstruction of venous drainage.

---

*This obsolete test was done to check for blockage of CSF in the spinal canal. Pressure was measured during a lumbar puncture with and without compression of the jugular veins. Normally, intracranial pressure is elevated when the jugular veins are compressed because venous blood stays in the cranium. If there is no blockage, this elevated pressure can be transmitted in part to the site of the lumbar puncture. In other instances this transmission is blocked (e.g., by a spinal tumor). The Queckenstedt test is now seldom performed because it is potentially hazardous and provides much less information than would be obtained from other equally invasive techniques such as myelography or non-invasive techniques such as CT or MRI scanning.

Arterioles in the brain are sensitive to changes in the partial pressures of the arterial blood gases, carbon dioxide and oxygen ($PaCO_2$ and PaO_2). They dilate when the $PaCO_2$ rises and when the PaO_2 falls, and constrict in the reverse situation. The arteriole thus serves to autoregulate (keep constant) brain cell metabolism.

Respiratory failure invariably involves an elevation of $PaCO_2$ and a fall in PaO_2. In this instance, the arteriolar reaction is to dilate, causing the vascular bed (blood volume) in the cranium to increase. In turn, intracranial pressure rises. At normal CSF pressures shown in Figs. 133–A and 134–A, a slight increase in the volume of the vascular bed has little effect on CSF pressure because it is buffered by the escape of CSF to the spinal canal. However, when the compensatory capacity of the CSF is exhausted, a small increase in intracranial volume (caused by an increased vascular bed) leads to a dramatic increase in CSF pressure (133–B, 134–B). This is frequently seen in patients with intracranial hemorrhage or cerebral tumor, who may suddenly deteriorate if a slight respiratory malfunction occurs. Examples of such respiratory disturbances include: epilepsy, unintentional swallowing of vomitus, relaxation of the tongue during impaired consciousness, retention of intratracheal secretions, complications of respiratory disease and central respiratory failure brought on by analgesics and sedatives. It deserves emphasis that these respiratory disturbances can cause serious damage in patients with brain disorders. Efforts should focus on the prevention and treatment of these disturbances, with the administration of oxygen being essential. During such administration (usually via the nose), there must be no obstruction of the glottis and intratracheal secretions must be cleared.

If intracranial pressure rises to approximate systemic blood pressure, cerebral blood vessels lose their autoregulatory capacity. Instead, they exhibit a flaccid dilation and progressive expansion (134–B) that precipitates even greater increases in intracranial pressure. If this vicious cycle continues, intracranial pressure eventually equals arterial pressure and brain death ensues, because the blood vessels become obliterated by external pressure.

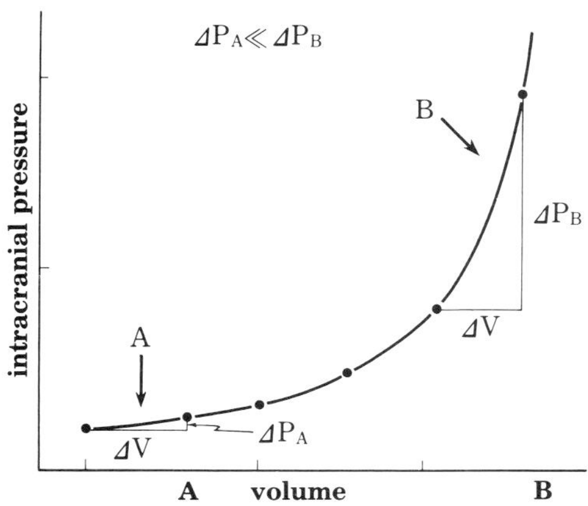

Fig. 133 The relationship between increased brain volume and intracranial pressure.
As brain volume linearly increases (e.g. A to B), intracranial pressure exponentially increases (P_A vs. P_B).

A normal autoregulation

arterial blood inflow

arterial blood pressure = 110 mmHg

pressure in the subarachnoid space = 10 mmHg

cerebral vascular resistance (present) autoregulation (intact)

cerebral vascular bed

CSF production

CSF absorption

venous blood outflow

B impaired autoregulation

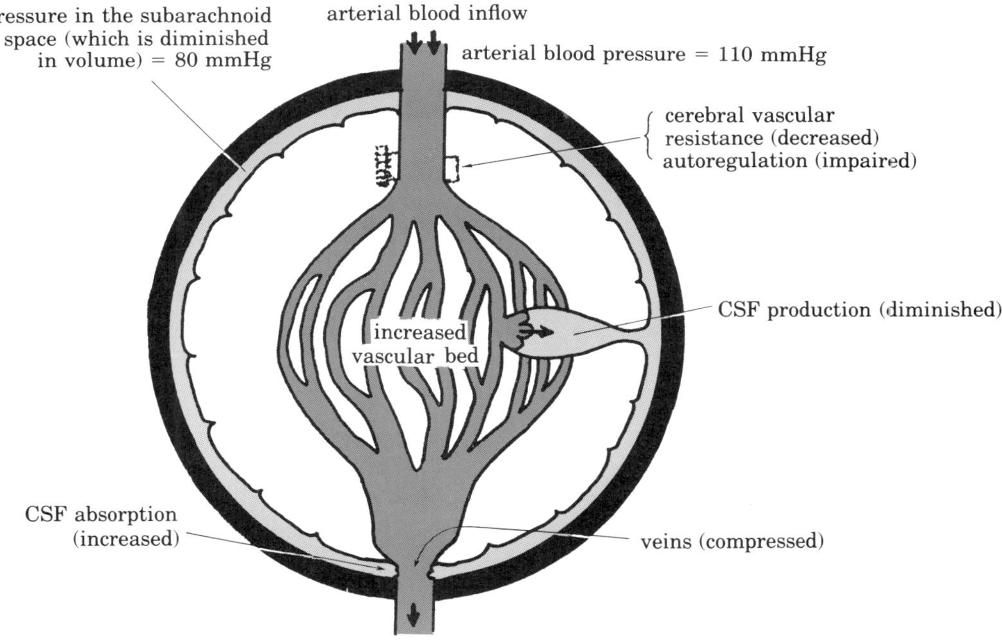

Fig. 134 Normal (A) and abnormal (B) blood vessels.

SPACE-TAKING LESIONS

If foreign material joins the cranial contents (e.g., a tumor, hematoma or abscess), it is inevitable that the intracranial pressure will rise over time. However, the first change is a compensatory movement of the pre-existing cranial contents, rather than an increase in the intracranial pressure (Fig. 135, 136–B). In this situation, since the brain substance is not reduced, the most important compensatory function is achieved by the movement of CSF. The volume of CSF in the cranium, including the ventricles, subarachnoid space and cisterns, is 100–150 ml. If some of this fluid is transferred to the subarachnoid space of the spinal cord then the growth can be accommodated and an increase in ICP will not occur (136–B). This is why an increased ICP is rarely seen in aged people, because more CSF occupies the space produced by atrophy of the brain. In this sense, their compensatory space is higher than that of the general population. It can be calculated that space-taking lesions of 100–150 ml should not cause increased ICP, but there is a delicate balance between the speed of CSF movement and the growth rate of a lesion. In the case of a benign tumor, ICP does not rise much until the tumor becomes quite large, because there is enough time for compensation to occur. A rapidly growing hematoma, however, can cause a remarkable increase in pressure even if its volume is less than 100 ml.

A. The normal situation

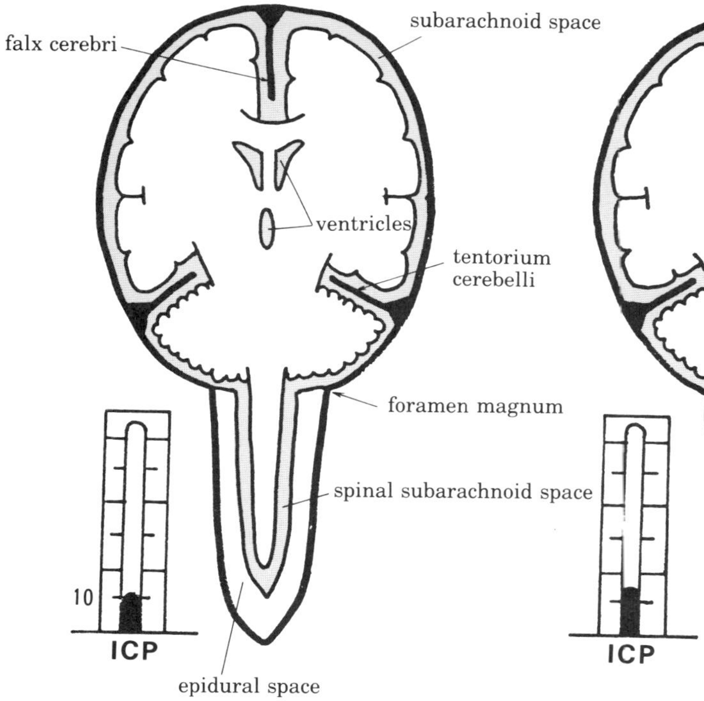

The ventricular CSF and the subarachnoid space play an important role in compensatory adjustments.

B. The beginning of compensation

ICP remains relatively normal, because some CSF in the ventricles and subarachnoid space of the affected side escapes in the subarachnoid space around the spinal cord.

Fig. 136 The enlargements of a space-taking lesion and its effect on intracranial pressure.

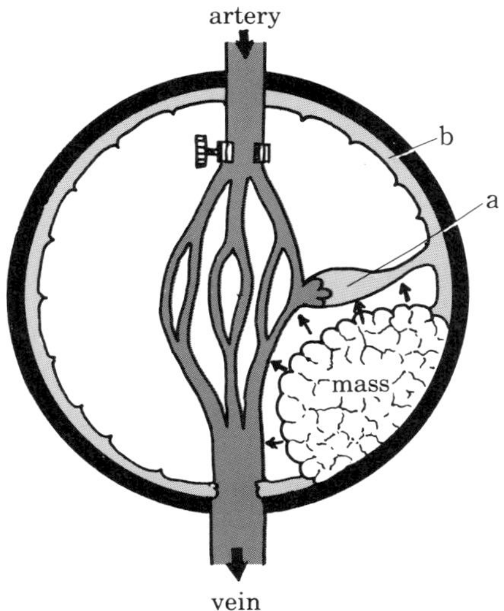

Fig. 135 A space taking lesion.
Note that the ventricle (a) and subarachnoid space (b) have suffered compensatory reductions.

C. The final stage of compensation

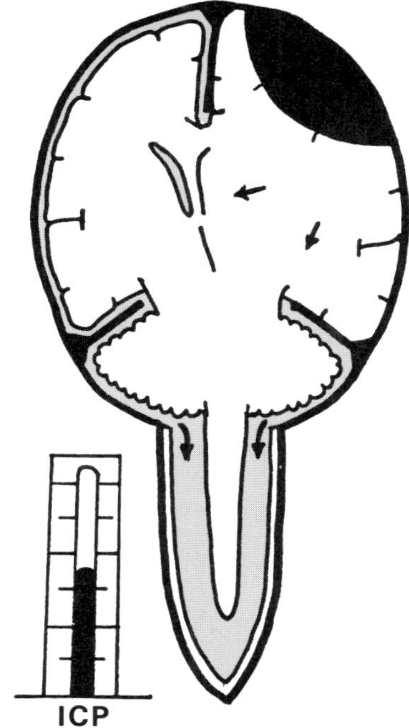

At this stage of CSF compensation, the brain begins to distort and shift and ICP starts to rise substantially.

D. Herniation

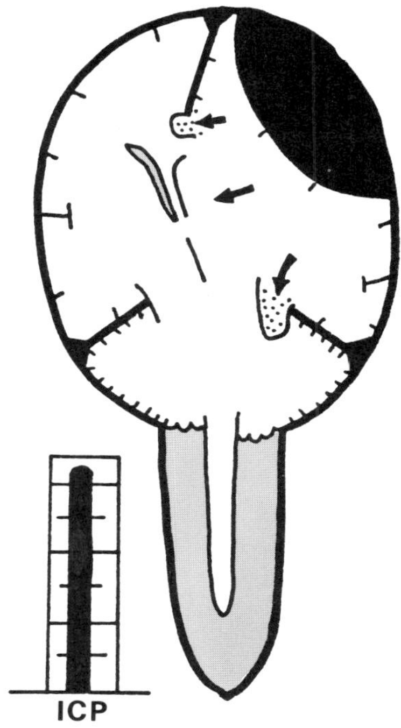

The CSF has almost completely transferred to the spinal cord. ICP has increased sufficiently to give rise to herniation, an extreme brain displacement.

CLINICAL SIGNS OF INCREASED INTRACRANIAL PRESSURE

When ICP rises, similar manifestations appear, regardless of the location and kind of brain lesion. If the symptoms or signs are not noted, the patient may die within a few days or weeks. Usually, there are three classical symptoms: 1) headache, 2) vomiting, 3) papilledema (choked disk). Except for papilledema, these symptoms are not restricted to cases of increased ICP, but are complained about in many other diseases. However, when they occur in combination, an increased ICP is immediately suspect and demands the most serious attention.

HEADACHE: The symptom is complained about more frequently in other conditions, but it is also the most frequent symptom of patients with increased ICP. Therefore, when a patient is examined for headache, the issue of increased ICP should always be addressed.

VOMITING: This usually accompanies headache; but not always. Vomiting as the chief complaint associated with increased ICP is more likely in children than in adults. Any disease which brings on an acute elevation of ICP (hematoma, etc.) is usually accompanied by a vomiting episode which occurs without warning. It is called projectile vomiting because of its severity.

CHOKED DISC (PAPILLEDEMA): The optic nerve is considered to be an extension of the brain. Out to the eye, it is completely covered by the dura mater and subarachnoid space. In cases of increased ICP, CSF is continuous with the subarachnoid space around the optic nerve, raising the pressure within the optic-nerve sheath. This compresses the axons and the central retinal vein as it enters the subarachnoid space (Fig. 137), leading to hyperemia and hemorrhage from the tributaries of this vein.

When a patient with papilledema complains of failing visual acuity, this is a sign of chronic increased ICP. As vision deteriorates, a secondary atrophy of the optic nerve often begins. Once initiated, this process usually leads to loss of vision, even if the original problem is reversed. Diplopia or double vision caused by increased ICP usually occurs due to an abducens nerve palsy.

DISTURBED CONSCIOUSNESS: When ICP is raised quickly by an extradural hematoma, a previously lucid patient often deteriorates without any external signs over a period of several hours. This loss of consciousness is thought to be due to a decreased blood circulation to the brain and dysfunction of the reticular formation of the brain stem. The evaluation procedure for acutely disturbed consciousness is described later.

In the case of a slow and gradual increase in ICP (over several weeks or months) caused by a supratentorial tumor, the patient first exhibits various personality changes including carelessness which gradually changes to indifference and depression, before finally becoming indecisive and then demented in the later stages.

ELEVATION OF BLOOD PRESSURE AND BRADYCARDIA: In the case of an acute increase in ICP, the perfusion pressure in the brain (systemic pressure minus intracranial pressure) is lowered. The systemic pressure then rises to send more blood (oxygen) to the brain, in an attempt to compensate for the increased ICP. The high blood pressure observed in this process is called the Cushing phenomenon. It is usually associated with a bradycardia caused by increased vagal activity. This bradycardia is a homeostatic mechanism, a well known symptom of increased ICP.

SYMPTOMS AND SIGNS OF INCREASED INTRACRANIAL PRESSURE IN INFANTS

When the ICP rises, infants rarely manifest behavior suggesting headache or visual disturbances. Rather, vomiting is the most frequent sign, particularly in the earliest stage. Several other clues include: 1) expansion of head-circumference, 2) protrusion of the fontanelles, 3) deviation of the external occipital protuberance (downward with a supratentorial, upward with an infratentorial mass), 4) engorgement of the scalp and facial veins and 5) Macewen's sign (percussion of the skull produces a resonant tone).

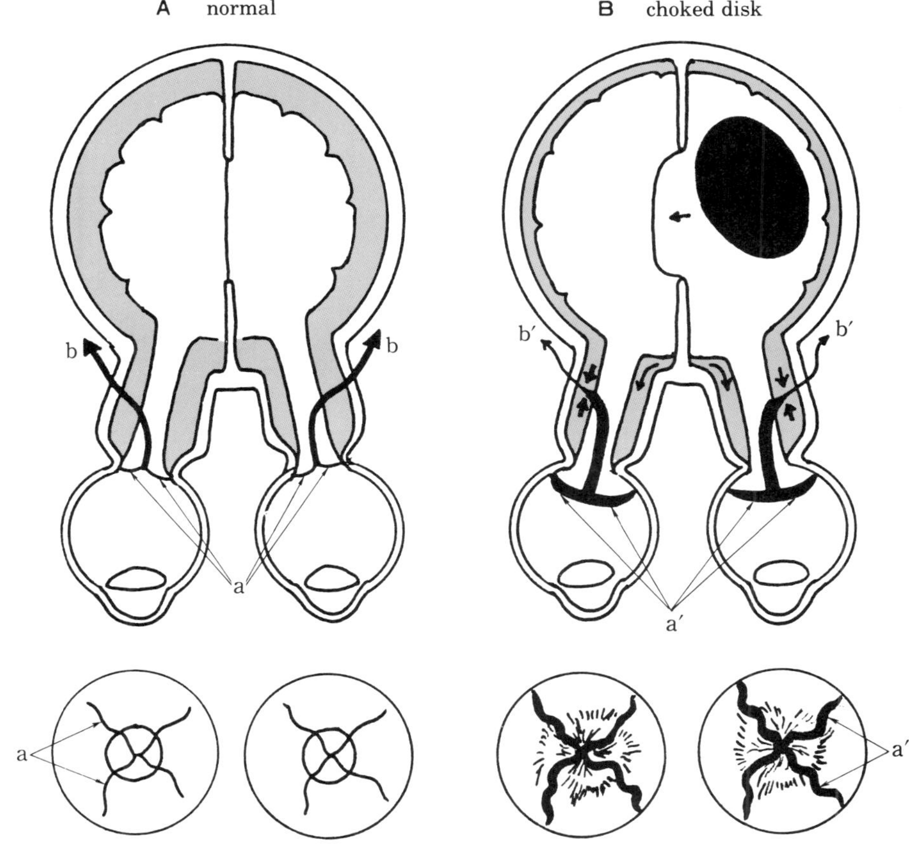

A. normal: The retinal central vein (a) runs within the optic nerve and then penetrates the subarachnoid space and emerges from the dura mater.

B. choked disk: A rise in ICP is transmitted to the subarachnoid space around the optic nerve. This compresses the central retinal vein at its point of penetration into the subarachnoid space. As a result the peripheral part of the vein retains blood and contributes towards an edematous papilla.

Fig. 137 The progress of choked disk (papilledema).

2. CEREBRAL HERNIATION

If space-occupying lesions continue to enlarge, ICP rises over time and the brain itself begins to distort (136–C). Brain substance in regions subjected to high pressure moves toward regions of low pressure. When this movement is sufficient to produce a symptom, it is called herniation. If it progresses to an irreversible state, it is called an incarcerated hernia (Fig. 136–D).

The intracranial space is divided into superior and inferior portions by the tentorium cerebelli and into left and right halves by the falx cerebri (Figs. 136–A, 138). When a space-occupying lesion occurs on one side of the supratentorial space, the increased mass extrudes below the medio-inferior part of the falx (138–A) and through the ipsilateral tentorial incisura (138–B). If the mass occurs in the infratentorial space, extrusion occurs downward through the foramen magnum, (142–B) and upward through the tentorial incisura (142–A). Thus, if treatment is not effected for a mass in the supratentorial space, a subfalcial herniation and a transtentorial herniation will occur (Fig. 138). If treatment is ineffective for a mass in the infratentorial space, an upward transtentorial herniation and a foraminal herniation will result (Fig. 142). Subfalcial herniation (cingulate herniation) (138–A) appears as a deviation of the anterior cerebral artery on carotid angiography or a lateral displacement of the lateral ventricle on head CT scan. It does not have marked symptoms. Upward transtentorial herniation (142–A), occasionally occurs when supratentorial pressure is abruptly reduced by ventricular drainage without an associated treatment for increased infratentorial pressure. It shows the same symptoms as a tentorial herniation (see below).

A cerebral herniation cannot be corrected if it is incarcerated. However, there are distinctive symptoms before this point. If the hernia is diagnosed in its early stage, then the possibility exists for a successful recovery.

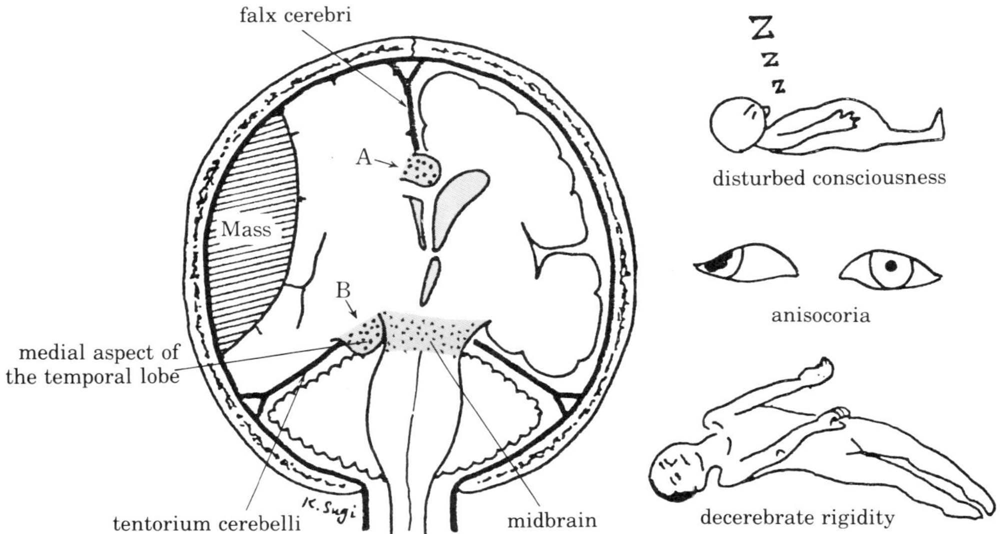

Fig. 138 Increased supratentorial ICP.
A. subfalcial herniation B. tentorial herniation

TENTORIAL HERNIATION
(synonyms: uncal herniation, temporal herniation)

Tentorial herniation is the final stage of increased supratentorial pressure. It leads to increased pressure and disturbances in the midbrain, which may be pressed against the opposite tentorial incisura, by an inferiorly herniated hippocampus or uncus (138–B, 140, 141).

Important early symptoms of tentorial herniation include:

1. An acute exacerbation of headache and vomiting
2. A progressive disturbance of consciousness
3. A slight anisocoria
4. A hemiparesis
5. A paresis of upward gaze.

If increased ICP is suspected, then specific and aggresive treatment should be provided immediately, even if the patient exhibits but a single and evanescent symptom. It is not acceptable to simply prescribe absolute rest and continue giving

Fig. 140 Kernohan's incisura.
A slowly developing tentorial herniation frequently gives rise to Kernohan's incisura (B). The midbrain is pushed to the margin of the contralateral tentorial incisura and damaged. The oculomotor nerve (A) is damaged on the affected (ipsilateral) side, and the pyramidal tract (C) on the contralateral side.

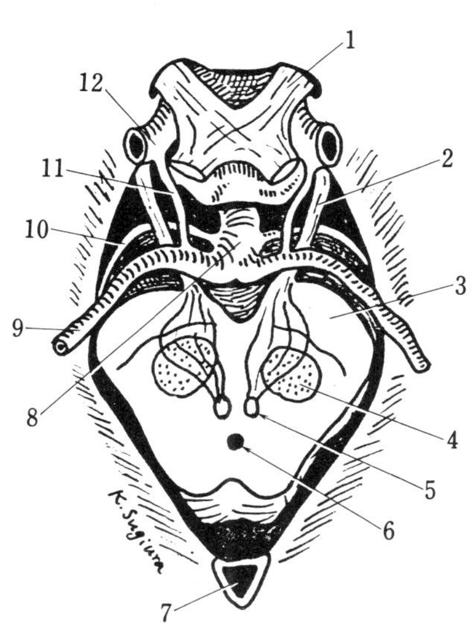

Fig. 139 Structures passing through the tentorial incisura.

1. optic nerve
2. oculomotor nerve
3. cerebral peduncle
4. red nucleus
5. oculomotor nucleus
6. cerebral aqueduct
7. straight sinus
8. basilar artery
9. posterior cerebral artery
10. superior cerebellar artery
11. posterior communicating artery
12. internal carotid artery

blood pressure depressants and oxygen.

Certain signs of severe midbrain dysfunction which include decerebrate rigidity, coma, and complete dilation of pupil are ominous prognostic signs regardless of prompt therapeutic intervention.

Anisocoria is due to oculomotor nerve compression (139–2, 140–A, 141) and frequently occurs on the same side as the affected hemisphere.

A hemiparesis on the contralateral side is a localizing sign of a space-occupying lesion. Compression and disturbance of the cerebral peduncle (139–3) on the same side may be caused by a temporal herniation. It exacerbates the contralateral hemiparesis. Of particular concern is a Kernohan's incisura deficit (140–B) which results in an ipsilateral hemiparesis. This is often seen when ICP rises slowly (e.g., in a chronic subdural hematoma). The contralateral cerebral peduncle is then progressively pressed against the tentorial incisura (Fig. 140). In this instance, if the side of the lesion is predicted by either the dilatation of the pupil or the hemiparesis and the predictions fail to show concordance, then there is less chance of an error if the pupil alone is used for localization.

Decerebrate rigidity can occur either unilaterally or bilaterally. During compression of the midbrain, this phenomenon is interpreted as a release from inhibition of muscle tone. This is a serious symptom, but sometimes, especially in children, recovery can be sufficent for a return to normal life.

A state of decortication is seen when a lesion includes the internal capsule. As in decerebrate rigidity, the lower extremities are maintained in an extended position, but, unlike decerebrate rigidity, the upper extremities are kept flexed at the elbow. The clinical significance of decortication resembles that of decerebrate rigidity, except that the prognosis of the former is far better than that of the latter.

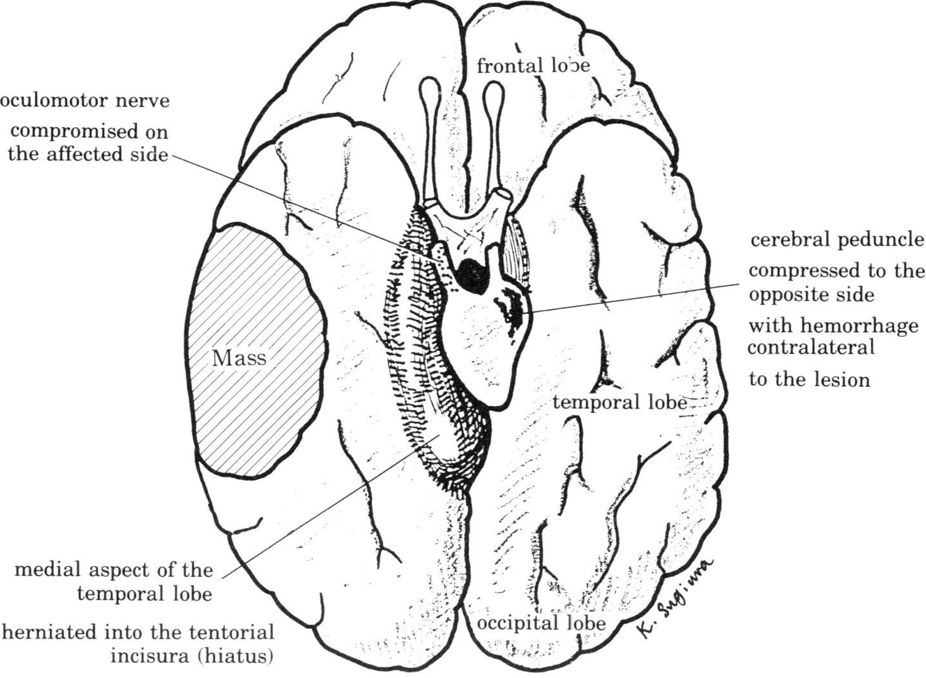

Fig. 141 A tentorial herniation.

FORAMINAL HERNIATION
(synonyms: cerebellar herniation, tonsillar herniation)

This herniation occurs when a cerebellar tonsil is trapped within the foramen magnum and the medulla oblongata is compressed (Fig. 142). In the case of an infratentorial lesion, the characteristic symptoms, like altered consciousness, do not always appear, but a sudden fatal arrest of respiration might occur. Therefore, in the case of a suspected infratentorial lesion, assessed by the combination of long-tract findings and cranial nerve palsies, extremely urgent treatment is necessary. Specific clues suggesting this problem include:

1. An abnormality of the depth and rhythm of breathing and, in particular, ataxic breathing (Fig. 142). This is caused by a disorder of the respiratory centers in the medulla. Such irregular breathing is different from that of Cheyne-Stokes respiration, which maintains a regular rhythm.
2. Frequent vomiting. This symptom is caused by stimulation of the vomiting center in the medulla.
3. Pain and stiffness of the neck.
4. An abnormal head position. Attention must be paid to a child who has an inclined head, in the attempt to avoid pain. (Tumors in infants and children are frequently infratentorial). By adopting such a head position, there is less stimulation of the meninges at the cranial base by a ptosed cerebellar tonsil.
5. Fulminant pain in the neck. A ptosed cerebellar tonsil is thought to involve cervical nerves.

The above mentioned symptoms, particularly 1, 2 and 3, are very important warning signs, and if overlooked, an arrest of breathing and death are certain. Treatment for an infratentorial lesion is even more urgent than for a tentorial herniation, in which death may be more protracted.

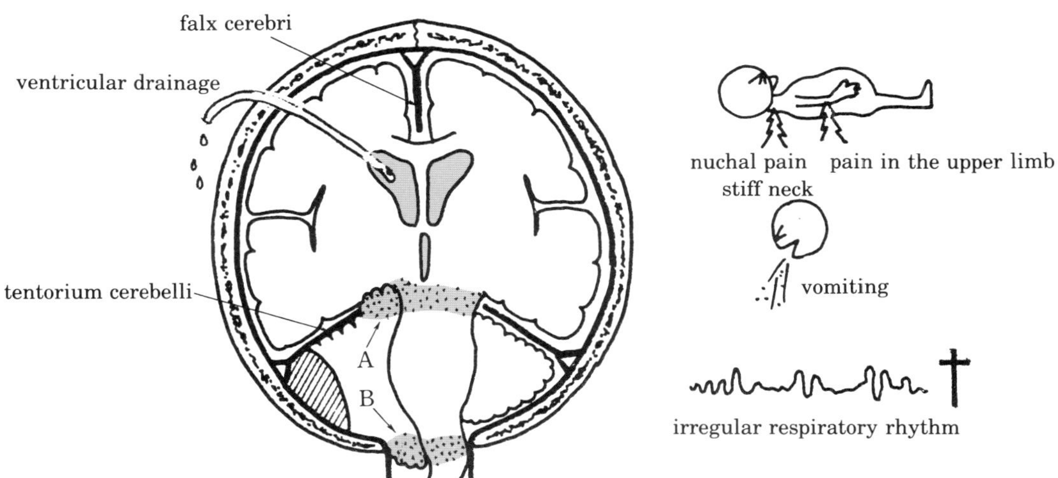

Fig. 142 A subtentorial compression.
A. upward transtentorial herniation B. foraminal (tonsillar) herniation

IMPORTANCE OF CONSTANT OBSERVATION

It is essential that the above-mentioned symptoms and signs be detected as soon as possible if treatment is to be successful. To achieve success it is first necessary to realize that potential candidates for herniation are those patients recovering from an intracranial operation, those with head trauma, intracerebral hemorrhage and other CNS masses. Second, patients with these conditions must be frequently examined for evidence of progressive deterioration, particularly: 1) level of consciousness, 2) pupillary function (anisocoria, light reflex), 3) frequency and regularity of respiration, 4) blood pressure and pulse rate and 5) motor and sensory dysfunction. The interval between observations depends on the state of the patient. As a general rule, intervals of 30 minutes are required for critical patients and 1–2 hours for potentially unstable cases such as those recovering from brain surgery. Through constant observation, many patients' lives can be saved, particularly if appropriate treatment is given to those suspected early of developing cerebral herniation.

3. MONITORING OF INTRACRANIAL PRESSURE

If increased ICP persists after removal of a hematoma or tumor, its continuous monitoring is required for a satisfactory outcome.

Although various devices are available to measure ICP, insertion of a catheter through a frontal perforation into the frontal horn (after Lundberg and colleagues, Fig. 143) is used most often. This procedure is often routine after neurosurgical operations. However, it may also be required during emergency situations. Sterilized perforators should be available in the emergency room, so that this procedure can be conducted immediately in this setting when appropriate. The pressure reading so obtained provides an important guide as to the effectiveness of treatment. If the ICP of a comatose patient is normal, then brain swelling is not causing the altered consciousness. If the increased ICP is treated and the patient remains comatose despite a reduced ICP, then a primary or secondary disorder of the brain-stem reticular formation or its projections is possible. If a reduction in ICP accompanies the recovery from neurological symptoms, then the patient may respond well to the normalization of the still-increased pressure. This catheter-insertion technique also has the advantage that drainage of CSF can be accomplished when necessary.

Fig. 144 shows an example of the continuous recording of ventricular pressure. Note the range of fluctuation of the ICP. Obviously, it is futile to make isolated pressure measurements by means of a lumbar puncture. CNS infection is always a potential complication of making an ICP measurement with a ventricular catheter. A lumbar puncture is potentially dangerous in this setting because of the brain herniation, and is contra-indicated.

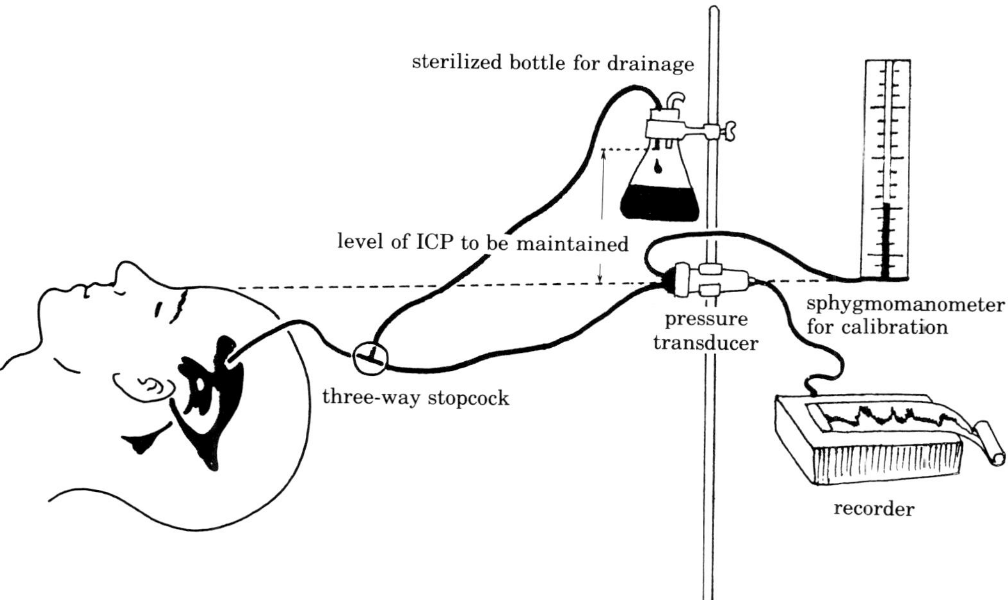

Fig. 143 The continuous monitoring of ICP.
The height of the transducer should be the same as the highest part of the head. The appropriate height of the drainage bottle is also shown. When the patient's head position is changed, the positions of the transducer and drainage bottle should be adjusted accordingly.

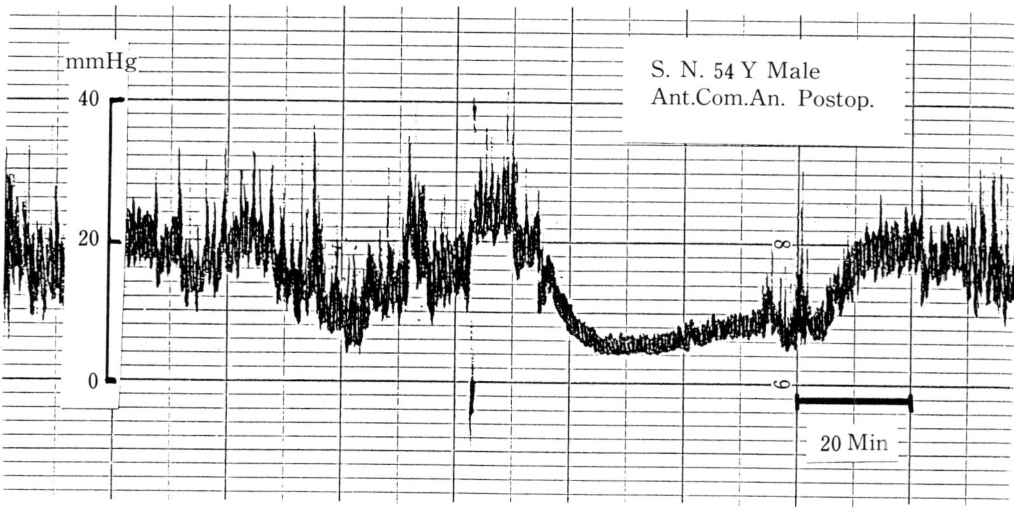

Fig. 144 An example of the continuous monitoring of intracranial pressure.
In patients with high cerebral pressure, the ICP fluctuates substantially. This illustrates the futility and the hazards of making momentary pressure measurements by means of a lumbar puncture.

4. IMPAIRMENT OF CONSCIOUSNESS

WHAT IS CONSCIOUSNESS?

The most important task in stabilizing a patient with an acute brain disturbance involves correct assessment of the degree of impairment of consciousness. A valuable clinical parameter of an acute brain dysfunction is a change in the level of consciousness. Although valuable information can be obtained from CT scanning and the continuous measurement of ICP, these procedures, although routine, cannot be utilized continuously for practical reasons. As a result, the constant monitoring of consciousness is important.

Physiological and anatomical mechanisms of consciousness have been studied intensively for several decades. A structure in the brain stem responsible for the maintenance of consciousness is called the reticular formation (Fig. 145) and in particular, a component called the ascending reticular activating system (ARAS). An organism's perceptions result, in part, from sensory input which projects via many different pathways to terminate in the cerebral hemispheres. These specific pathways are major avenues for sensory perception. These and other non-specific pathways, all provide collateral input to the ARAS which processes it and sends information via diffuse projections to the entire cerebral cortex. In so doing, the ARAS primes the cerebrum to maintain an appropriate level of consciousness. The ARAS extends from the thalamus to the medulla. Its more rostral component (above the midbrain) is more important for consciousness than its lower part (caudal to the pons). For example, consciousness might not be lost in "locked-in syndrome", which is caused by a widespread pontine disorder.

EVALUATION OF CONSCIOUSNESS: THE EDINBURGH COMA SCALE

Techniques for an objective evaluation of altered consciousness have been available for over two decades. One is the Edinburgh coma scale 1 (E1CS), which classifies the reactions of patients with impaired consciousness into seven divisions by applying three levels of sensory stimulation to the patient, including: 1) a simple question, 2) a simple command if there is no answer to the simple question and 3) a strong noxious stimulus if there is no reaction to the command. It has been shown many times that E1CS provides a high correlation between the patient's level of consciousness and the subsequent prognosis (Table 13).

In 1974, the Glasgow coma scale (GCS) was developed in the United Kingdom, followed by the 3–3–9 scale in Japan. The latter had too large an inter-observer error to provide a reliable evaluation. The GCS has the advantage that three key reactions of the patient, eye opening, speech and movement of the extremities are evaluated and described separately. This approach is based on the belief that functions controlled by different CNS systems should be evaluated separately. However, a limitation of the GCS scoring system is that the evaluated functions are not weighted and the numerical scores denoting the extent of altered consciousness are not as meaningful as those provided by the E1CS system.

Table 13. EDINBURCH COMA SCALE (E1CS, 1973) AND PATIENT PROGNOSIS

RESPONSE TO STIMULUS SCORE	DEATH	SURVIVALS DISTURBED	SURVIVALS SOUND	TOTAL NO. OF CASES
0. normal responses to natural stimuli	14(9)	24(16)	116(75)	154
1. answering a loud and simple question	18(15)	26(22)	75(63)	119
2. reacting to a loud and simple command	18(14)	53(41)	59(45)	130
3. purposeful responses of the extremities to strong noxious stimulation	69(53)	32(25)	29(22)	130
4. flexion of the extremities to the same noxious stimulus	82(57)	36(25)	26(18)	144
5. extension of the extremities to the same noxious stimulus	82(57)	7(9)	3(4)	75
6. no reaction to noxious stimulation	65(87)	7(9)	3(4)	75

Numbers in parenthesis denote %. E1CS levels and patient prognoses correlate significantly for both mortality rates ($r=0.938$, $P<0.01$) and survival ($r=0.988$, $P<0.01$). This suggests that the E1CS is ordinal.

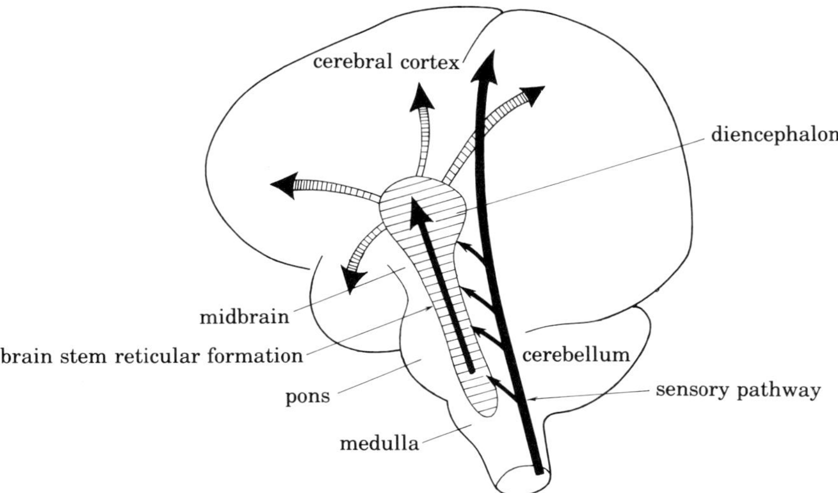

Fig. 145 Pathways for awareness.

IMPROVED EDINBURGH COMA SCALE

An improved E1CS, called the E2CS (Table 14), was recently developed. It is based on the same principle as the E1CS but is less prone to inter-observer error. Its use is currently increasing.

An examiner firstly asks two questions loudly, "How old are you?" and "What month is it now?" The examiner marks the answers correct or not, regardless of the style of answering, which may be verbal, writing on paper or nodding. For two correct answers, the best score [1] is assigned. If one of the two answers is correct, the score is [2] and if both answers are incorrect or not understandable, the score is [3].

If there are no responses to the questions, the second step involves presenting two vocal stimuli. The examiner gives loud commands, "clench and open your hands!" and "Open and close your eyes!" Correct responses are scored with a [4], one correct response with [5] and two incorrect responses with [6]. Incorrect responses include clenching but not opening the hands, and opening but not closing the eyes. If the patient attempts the correct responses but fails in their execution, then the score [6] is again assigned.

If no responses are obtained in the second step, strong noxious stimulation is applied as a third step. The sternum is rubbed strongly or the skin around the arm pit is pinched. The motor responses to this noxious stimulation is assigned three scores. If the patient tries to drive away the examiners' hands, the score is [7]. If the arms and legs are flexed, the score is [8] and if the extremities are extended, the score is [9]. No movement of the extremities to strong noxious stimulation is scored as [10].

Repelling motions by the patient suggest that the cerebrum can perceive pain and identify its source and cause. If the patient is not successful in removing the examiner's pain-eliciting actions, but still moves the hands to the site of noxious stimulation, then the score [7] can be assigned, because the patient is aware of the overall situation. In contrast, flexion of the extremities is considered a component of a spinal reflex concerned with escape from adverse stimulation. Finally, extension of the extremities is a pathological response, seen sometimes in decerebrate rigidity.

There are two important aspects to the E2CS procedure. First, continuous and maximum stimulation is necessary. Even in the case of normal subjects, the eyes may not open during deep sleep unless commanded to do so by a rather loud voice. Weak stimuli cause errors in the estimation of the level of consciousness. A second consideration is that the examiner must select the best response among those exhibited by the patient. For example, a patient who is able to state his age might not be able to respond to an eye open-close command. Other patients might reveal verbally that they are being subjected to noxious stimulation but lack the means to make appropriate motor responses. In these instances, the verbal responses reveal the level of consciousness. In hemiplegics, the affected extremity cannot move and it would be futile to command or stimulate it to do so as an index of consciousness.

Table 14. THE IMPROVED EDINBURGH COMA SCALE (E2CS, 1978)

STIMULUS	RESPONSE	SCORE
Loud question:	Two correct answers	1
{What month is it now?	One correct answer	2
How old are you?}	Two incorrect answers	3
Loud command:	Two correct reactions	4
{Clench your hands, and open.	One correct reaction	5
Open your eyes, and close.}	Two incorrect reactions	6
Strong noxious stimulation	Driving-away-action	7
	Flexion of extremities	8
	Extension of extremities	9
	No reaction	10

(It should be remembered that the scores are based on the best responses to maximum stimuli.)

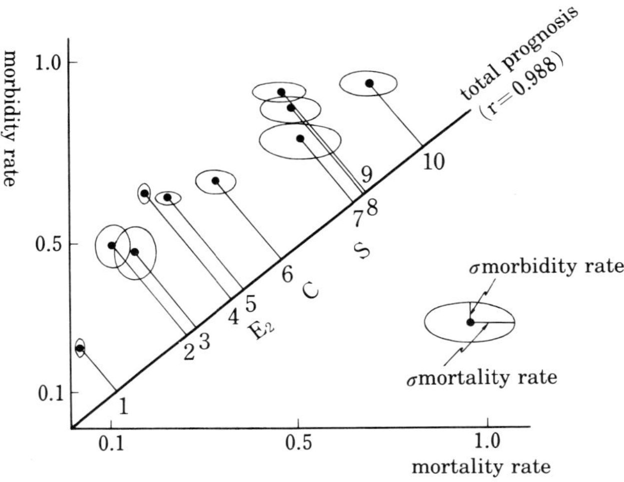

Fig. 146 E2CS scaling.

SCALING CONSIDERATIONS (Fig. 146)

While a variety of scaling procedures other than E1CS and E2CS are now being used in various clinics, there is still no consensus on the criteria required for effectively scaling levels of consciousness. Clearly, the evaluation of different scaling techniques is an important consideration, but to date, it has been considered only by us (K.S.) for the E1CS and E2CS and by Jenett for the GCS.

The inter-observer errors of doctors and nurses are few for E1CS and E2CS when compared to the 3–3–9 and the GCS scales. If there is appropriate team-work between nurses and doctors, then experienced doctors can rely more on the scores furnished by nurses and inexperienced doctors. This is the reason why the E2CS is recommended for use by the full medical staff, including nurses charged with the responsibility of observing patients with brain disorders throughout the night.

SYNDROMES RELATED TO IMPAIRED CONSCIOUSNESS (Fig. 147)

Impaired consciousness is not restricted to neurosurgical patients. It is also related to internal medicine and general surgery. Examples include hepatic and diabetic coma, acute drug intoxication and coma after shock or anoxia. Each of these has distinctive features, but space constraints preclude their descriptions here. Rather, some brief descriptions are now provided about pathological conditions which share symptoms in common with impaired consciousness and brain death.

1. APHASIA

It is difficult to evaluate the level of consciousness of the aphasic patient. Usually, the examination makes use of verbal questions and commands. When the patient has a global aphasia, their responses may suggest impaired consciousness, particularly confusion. In the future, the analysis of the electroencephalogram (EEG) and evoked potentials should prove helpful with this kind of patient.

2. DEMENTIA AND PSYCHOSIS

Serious dementia, hysterical fits, profound depression and the catatonia of schizophrenia are often confused with impaired consciousness. Initially, it is important not to simply discount these patients as being psychiatric. Even if psychiatric disorders are a possibility, efforts must be made to exclude structural and metabolic disorders by obtaining a head CT scan, EEG, lumbar puncture and appropriate blood tests.

3. LOCKED-IN SYNDROME

When a lesion is present in the ventral pons, a paralysis of movement of the extremities and a bulbar palsy will occur. In this instance, impaired consciousness might be mistakingly diagnosed, because the patient cannot express their intentions with speech or movement of the extremities. However, careful testing reveals that such patients can communicate by perpendicular eye movements or by blinking.

4. COMA VIGIL (AKINETIC MUTISM)

Patients with coma vigil exhibit symptoms like those seen after chronic impaired consciousness. The patient manifests the appearance of being awake. When the eyes are open, they can be seen to be conjugately moving. They may turn their heads toward sound. This condition can be considered a profound dementia with no cognitive processing at the cortical level, but with preservation of brain stem reflex functions.

5. PERSISTENT VEGETATIVE STATE (PVS)

This term is used for patients in a chronic state of impaired consciousness, including the coma vigil described above. When three or four weeks have passed after acute brain trauma, the patient might occasionally recover the ability to open the eyes, but evidence of consciousness is still lacking. The term, PVS, is a term for all states involving chronically impaired consciousness including, for example, protracted coma and "apallic syndrome". Many neurosurgery wards have a few patients in a PVS. Often, they have been abandoned by their families and have been comatose for years. This is currently a very emotional issue due to advances in technology, and the incidence of these patients is on the rise. Their exorbitant medical

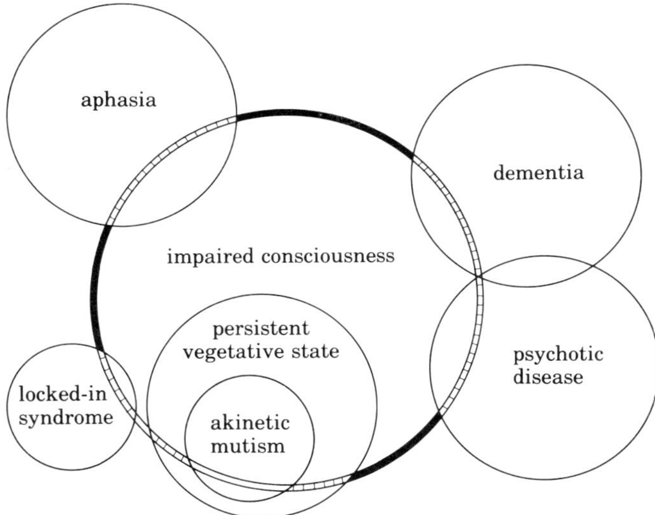

Fig. 147 Impaired consciousness and related symptoms.

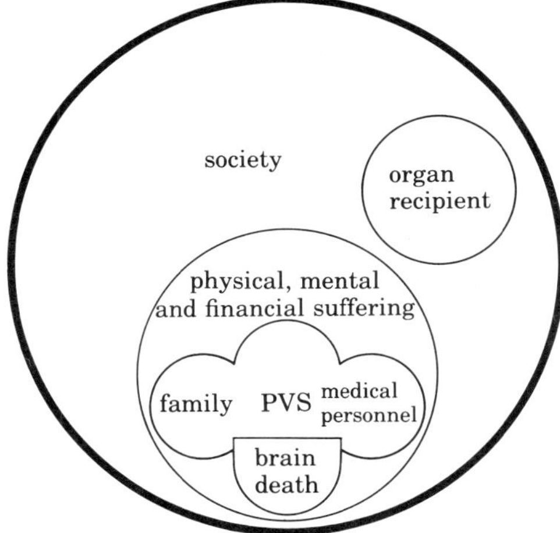

Fig. 148 The interplay between long-term impaired consciousness, brain death and society.

expenses are creating a major societal problem, which will require courageous acts that accommodate patient, family and social needs.

6. BRAIN DEATH (Fig. 148)

Brain death, as a permanent state, was not an issue when medical science was in its infancy. The definition of brain death in Japan and most other advanced countries involves: 1) deep coma, 2) mid-position and fixed pupils, 3) absence of autonomous breathing, 4) absence of brain stem reflexes 5) no movement in response to painful stimuli, 6) electrocerebral silence (by EEG) and 7) continuation of signs 1–6 for 6 hours.

The definition, evaluation and disposition of brain death cases are particularly challenging in modern civilized societies, including the needs of many people awaiting organ transplants. It is now up to medical philosophers to provide society with rational guidelines for handling this unfortunate condition.

INDEX

A

B

C

D

E

F

G

H

T

U

V

W

J.S. REYNOLDS COMMUNITY COLL